Praise for Food for Eyes

The attention to detail is amazing. I think this book will be a valuable resource. Some professionals seem to function in a bubble in that they find it difficult to embrace perspectives outside the parameters of their specialty. I think this book will go a long way to bridge that gap.
Katharina Prior, colleague.

Ms Mitchell has created a very easy to read book with lots of commonsense information, still controversial in some circles, for eye health and healthy eating.
Alan Smith, B. Pharm.

Food for Eyes is an excellent book and a must read for those with failing vision. JB Mitchell points out the value of eating a diet with the correct balances of nutrition, of vitamins, antioxidants, fats, Omega 3 and 6, and avoidance of processed food. She advises regular exercise, no smoking, minimal alcohol, and avoidance of obesity and its accompanying diabetes.

The book is well-researched, with her 68 references. Those readers without a scientific background may find part of the book a little heavy reading.

W.D. Walker, FRACS OAM

I seized on some of the information useful for "ailing vision" and support all Ms Mitchell proposes for a healthy life, for the elderly in particular. The print is suited to readers with diminished vision. The cover is most attractive.

Angela Jones PhD

A brief personal introduction as to how this book came about is convincing as to why one should read more.

The first chapter looks at a concise and straight forward structure and functioning of the eye. Mitchell then lists 22 of the common eye diseases. What is so relevant here, is her focus on the two most common eye problems associated with the ageing process.

The chapter on "things" that can damage your eyes is really a whole lot more than eyes only and is more concentrated on *quality* of life. Similarly the, "Foods that can Damage your Eyes" are also relevant to every day good health; such as sugar, starch, soy and fats and oils. The latter is given a very thorough factual chapter, on its own.

The chapter on, "Antioxidants to the rescue" is particularly related to our eyes and therefore invaluable. The author lists some twenty foods that help maintain healthy eyes before moving on to "supplements", particularly vitamins and minerals. Exercise and food together (with a few warnings about the latter and also about autoimmune disorders), complete Mitchell's book.

This brief review would not be complete without the mention of the 'friendly' size font and the simple little sketches throughout. Sixty-eight references reflect the hours of research tucked away in the pages of "Food for Eyes".

Yes, we all value our eyes as our most important asset. Not to be taken for granted as so many of us, especially as we grow older, know. An extremely worthwhile book.

Lorraine Taylor, book reviewer for Good Reads.

Food for Eyes: Nutrients for ailing vision

JB Mitchell Dip. Clin. Nutr.

A Large Print Book from Lakehouse

Published by Lakehouse Publishing
Lake Macquarie City, Australia.

© 2020 JB Mitchell.
© Illustrations by Kira and Tane Mitchell.
© Cover illustration by Nick Handlinger.

The rights of JB Mitchell as author of this work have been asserted. Apart from use as permitted under the Australian Copyright Act of 1968, no part of this book may be produced by any means without prior written permission from the author.

ISBN: 9780648497646 (pbk)

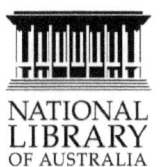

A catalogue record for this work is available from the National Library of Australia

Printed in Australia in Verdana font size 12.

Author's contact: jan.mitchell2021@gmail.com

Web: writingsfromjanmitchell.com

Titles from this author available from the publisher, 10 Rosemary Row, Rathmines, NSW 2283.
Also available as digital print on demand from all major booksellers and ebook retailers.

Contents

Figures and Tables	iii
Introduction	v
One: The parts of your eye	1
Two: Some common eye ailments	5
Three: Things that might damage your eyes	15
Four: Foods that could protect your eyes	29
Five: More about fats, oils	43
Six: Antioxidants	57
Seven: Foods to avoid	75
Eight: Blood supply to your eyes	89
Nine: In summary - How to proceed	91
Acknowledgements	105
References	107
Index	117
About the author	127

Figures and Tables

1. The eye — 1
2. Short and long focus — 3
3. Essential fatty acid content in land animals — 38
4. Oils and fats – Type of fat content — 51
5. Unpaired electrons become free radicals — 55
6. Chemical molecules belong to either left or right handed forms — 61
7. Cellular binding sites are often compared to keys and keyholes — 62
8. Lutein and Zeaxanthin in Foods — 66
9. Lutein content in green vegetables — 67

Introduction

I have written this book because I want to share with others how I have improved my vision when the prognosis was for it to worsen until I was virtually blind. Food, supplements and exercise are key factors in ameliorating eye disease.

When I was diagnosed with age related macular degeneration (AMD) about twelve years ago, I was terrified of the prognosis that I would lose my vision. Being an author, I felt that to lose my vision would be worse than to lose my ability to hear. I think it would be the opposite way round if I were a musician.

For most of my adult life I have had an interest in nutrition. This interest is shared with my husband and I decided to formalise my nutritional knowledge in the 1990s by adding a post graduate diploma in clinical nutrition to my two degrees and various other diplomas.

My husband and I both suffer from autoimmune disorders, as does one of our sons, and we have sought ways to mitigate these problems without drugs. It was natural therefore that I would do the same for macular degeneration.

On a visit to my optometrist, I saw a product which was approved by the optometry world as beneficial for eyes. The ingredients included lutein, zeanthaxin and synthetic vitamin E.

At that time I was taking a product from a large Australian supplement company. That product, with macular on its label, had provided no improvement to my eyes. However, in a small bottle beside it on the shelf, I noticed a product called *Lutein Defence*. As well as lutein it included zeanthaxin, but no vitamin E. Weren't lutein and zeanthaxin the same substances that optometric research had shown was beneficial? I was already taking natural vitamin E.

When I started taking *Lutein Defence* every day, I felt like my right eye was seeing the world through a gauze curtain. I was using my left eye more and more, but the problem was encroaching there too.

I started researching lutein and zeaxanthin, both antioxidants. Then I heard about anthocyanins, yet another form of antioxidant that was purported to be good for the eyes and brain. I found that red cabbage and blueberries contained high amounts. Once I started eating red cabbage and later blueberries every day, the gauze curtain began to withdraw. Slowly, I began to see the world almost clearly again.

Whilst the curtain has been pulled, the macular degeneration has not gone altogether. The lines on the test grid (Amsler Grid) are still wobbly. It is probable that the damage caused to my macula will never disappear.

In the meantime, I am delighted to be able to see the world more clearly today than for the past decade and to be able to continue my writing, especially to be able to spread the word about what might help other eye conditions.

It is my hope that by sharing my knowledge and experience with you, you will be able to take control of your eye condition in a manner that may help to ward off serious eyesight problems.

JB Mitchell, BA, MEd, Dip. Tchg., Dip. Rem. Ther., Post Graduate Diploma in Clinical Nutrition.

Disclaimer:

The advice given in this book is general in nature. More recent research may indicate other approaches for eye care.

If you take medications for serious health conditions, consult your GP, specialist and pharmacist before making changes to your diet and supplements.

One

The Parts of Your Eye

If you want to understand what is happening to your eyes as time passes, you might want to know the basics of eye anatomy. You might need to identify, at least, your pupil, lens, iris, retina, macula and optic nerve.

Figure 1: The Eye

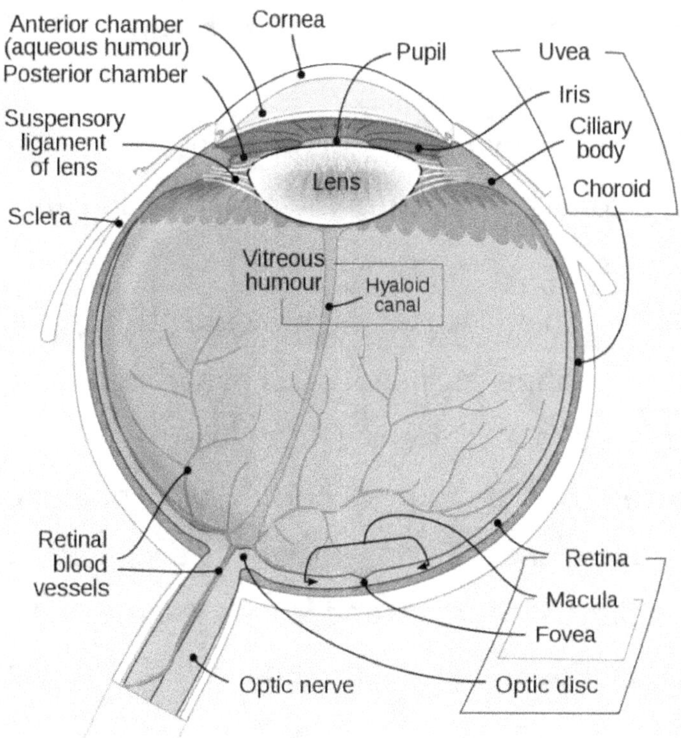

Image copied from:
https://commons.wikimedia.org/w/index.php?curid=1597930

Definitions of the parts of your eyes

These are definitions of the parts of your eyes shown in the diagram:[1]

Cornea – The clear skin that covers the front of your eye is as clear as glass and contains no blood vessels.

Sclera – The tough skin that surrounds most of the outside of the eyeball is known as the "white" of the eye.

Iris – The coloured part of your eye (blue, brown, green...) is the iris that controls the amount of light that enters your eye.

Pupil – The hole in the iris that lets light into your eye becomes tiny in bright sunlight and larger in darkness.

Lens – This focuses light onto the retina. It changes shape as needed to ensure the "picture" on the retina is as clear as possible.

Retina –This is your camera. The retina receives the light signals from which you see. Your retina has cells called rods and cones (named for their shape). Rods see black and white; cones see colour.

Each eye has about 120 million rods and 7 million cones! Together, they're responsible for changing the received light through the lens of your eye into impulses. Those impulses are then carried to the brain along your optic nerve.

Blind spot – This is a tiny spot on your retina, which isn't sensitive to light because it has no rods or cones. This is the spot where the optic nerve joins the retina.

Optic nerve – This nerve transmits the electrical messages from the retina to your brain.

Macula – This lies in the centre of your retina. It produces your central vision which enables you to read, drive, and perform other activities requiring fine, sharp, straight-ahead vision. [1]

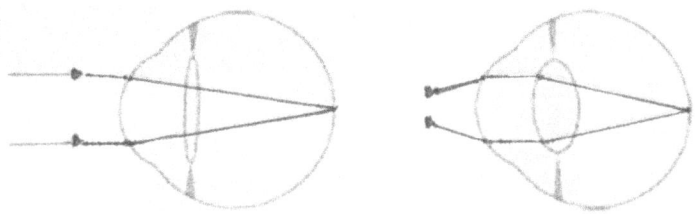

Long sight and short sight

After light enters your pupil, it hits the lens – which focuses those light rays on the retina at the back of your eyeball. The retinal nerve sends the signal from the rods and cones there to your brain, which interprets the images. [1]

Two

Some Common Eye Diseases

Without intervention, eye diseases might lead to blindness. These are the most common eye diseases that affect us as we age and where nutrition and exercise can help.

If you experience any of the following, you need to seek help from an optometrist. If the condition proves serious, you will be referred to an eye specialist (ophthalmologist).[2.]

- Change in iris colour
- Crossed eyes
- Dark spot in the centre of your field of vision
- Difficulty focusing on near or distant objects
- Double vision
- Dry eyes with itching or burning
- Episodes of cloudy vision
- Excess discharge or tearing
- Eye pain
- Floaters or flashers
- Growing bump on the eyelid
- Halos (coloured circles around lights) or glare
- Hazy or blurred vision
- Inability to close an eyelid
- Loss of peripheral vision

- Redness around the eye
- Spots in your field of vision
- Sudden loss of vision
- Trouble adjusting to dark rooms
- Unusual sensitivity to light or glare
- Veil obstructing vision
- Wavy or crooked appearance to straight lines

Cataracts and AMD (macular degeneration) are the most common eye problems in aging people.

Cataract

A cataract is a condition that causes clouding of the eye's lens as we age, which leads to a decrease in vision. Cataracts are the most common cause of eyesight problems as we age.

"Cataract surgery involves removing the eye's clouded lens and replacing it with a clear synthetic version. These days it is a very quick outpatients' operation, performed under local anaesthesia and people are back to their normal lives within days. The success rate is high, and the rate of vision-threatening complications is relatively low.

"For people with cataracts, the decision whether to have surgery may be easy to make. However, two additional decisions might be more difficult: when to have surgery and what type of lens implant to get," says Dr. Laura Fine, an ophthalmologist at the Harvard-affiliated Massachusetts General Hospital.

"While cataracts occur more often in people with osteoporosis, the relationship with calcium is not causal. Some people think calcium deposits are the cause of the clouding of the lens. This is not so. However, while too much or too little calcium in the diet can be linked to vision problems like cataract, cataracts are made of clumps of protein that form on the lens, not calcium deposit," Laura Fine says in a Harvard Health Newsletter.[3.]

In 2010, also in a Harvard Health Newsletter, Celeste Robb-Nicholson, M.D. said, "The cells of the lens are composed of water and protein arranged in a way that keeps the lens clear. For reasons that aren't fully understood, the protein molecules may clump together and start to cloud the lens. This is the beginning of a cataract. The effect has been likened to cooking an egg white.

"You may not notice anything at first, but cataracts typically progress, becoming denser or clouding more of the lens and blurring vision. Eventually, vision may be so severely affected that surgery is needed to remove the lens and replace it with an artificial one. Cataracts usually form in both eyes but may not progress at the same rate or affect vision equally in both eyes.

"We know how to treat cataracts, but we don't know much about why they develop. Aging is obviously a factor — possibly because of changes in the chemical composition of the lens or possibly because of normal wear and tear. Most people develop some lens opacity, or clouding, by the age of 60. Other risk factors include injury to the eye, previous eye surgery, diabetes, use of corticosteroid drugs, and having a family member with cataracts. Many studies have implicated smoking and drinking as well. And a study suggests that hormone therapy may increase the risk. Cataracts also seem to be more common in people who have had long-term exposure to sunlight.

"We don't know if avoiding or treating these risk factors will prevent a cataract from forming. But it can only do you good to refrain from smoking, moderate your alcohol consumption, and protect your eyes from sunlight with hats and sunglasses.

"Evidence on the role of diet in cataract prevention is mixed. Some experts believe that antioxidant vitamins might help prevent cataracts by getting rid of molecules called free radicals, which may trigger or fuel protein clumping. However, despite several studies, there is no convincing evidence yet that vitamin supplements prevent or slow cataract growth. In a 2008 *Archives of Ophthalmology* study, researchers found that women ages 50 to 79 whose diets were rich in lutein and zeaxanthin had fewer cataracts. These phytochemicals are abundant in dark green leafy vegetables such as spinach, kale, Swiss chard, watercress, and dandelion greens. But these vegetables contain many other healthy substances, so it's not clear whether lutein and zeaxanthin are responsible for the eye benefits."[4.]

Diabetic Retinopathy

Diabetic Retinopathy is a serious complication of diabetes. Diabetes is the condition when insulin production is unable to keep up with the blood's demand to modify sugar (in the form of glucose) for use as energy in your cells. A poorly-balanced diet with too much refined sugar, flour, seed oils and insufficient fresh vegetables may, among other things, lead to being overweight which is related to the development of diabetes and consequently, diabetic retinopathy.[5.]

Dry Eye

Dry eye is a condition in which a person does not have enough secretions to lubricate and nourish the eye. Tears are necessary for maintaining the health of the front surface of the eye and for providing clear vision. Dry eye is a common and often chronic problem, particularly in older adults.

It might be a side effect of other eye conditions, a side effect of some drugs, or a blockage of the glands which secrete moisture into the eyes. As the eyes become dry, they can feel itchy or gritty, as if there's something in the eye. The eyes may be red, and if they're sore they may be watery, which can cause vision to become blurry.[6.]

It is important to keep the eyes clean by using a fresh, damp cotton bud to clear the corners of the eyes after sleep.

If the eyelids become swollen, wring out a clean cloth in warm water and hold over the closed eyelids. It is possible the warmth will free up any sticky blockage in the secretory glands. [Ibid.] If these remedies don't help, you will need help from a specialist.

Glaucoma

Glaucoma, one of the leading causes of blindness for people over the age of 60, is a group of four eye conditions that can damage the optic nerve, the health of which is vital for good vision. This damage is sometimes caused by abnormally high pressure in the eye. Glaucoma tends to run in families.[7, 8.]

High blood pressure can cause damage to the retina and result in **hypertensive retinopathy**, which is damage to the retina and retinal circulation.[9.] However, high pressure in the eye is only sometimes linked to very high blood pressure, and low blood pressure may result in poor oxygen supply to the eye, which might also lead to retinal damage (glaucoma). [Ibid.]

I strongly recommend exercise as good medicine for all body health, including eyes. However, you must exercise with your head higher than your heart if you have high pressure in your eyes.

Age-related macular degeneration or AMD

AMD is when a yellowish-brown plaque called drusen results in blurred or little vision in the centre of the visual field.[10.] There are two main variations of AMD: dry and wet. Dry AMD is more common.

"The most advanced stage of dry age-related macular degeneration is known as **geographic atrophy**, in which areas of the macula waste away (atrophy), resulting in severe vision loss. Dry age-related macular degeneration typically affects vision in both eyes, although vision loss often occurs in one eye before the other."[11.]

"Dry AMD may progress and cause central vision loss without becoming wet AMD.

"[Wet AMD occurs in] 10 to 15 percent of affected individuals.... The wet form is characterized by the growth of abnormal, fragile blood vessels underneath the macula. These vessels leak blood and fluid, which damages the macula and makes central vision appear blurry and distorted. The wet form of age-related macular degeneration is associated with severe vision loss that can worsen rapidly." [10]

Like many modern diseases, the incidence of AMD parallels the growth of the modern processed food industry. The changed intake from animal fats to vegetable oils like industrial seed oils, increased sugar consumption and the change from cold-rolled grains to modern flour milling techniques has led to a loss of nutrients in our food, increased inflammation in our bodies and the consequent development of many diseases.[12]

Unfortunately, vision loss in wet AMD through loss of retinal pigment epithelial cells and photoreceptors cannot be regained by diet, says Dr Chris Knobbe (Ophthalmologist and founder of Cure AMD Foundation) on his website.

The Mayo clinic claims, "[N]o one knows exactly what causes dry macular degeneration." [10]

Many eye conditions can be linked to modern diet, and also to repeated excessive glare.

"Healthy vision may seem like a distant concern when you're young. But if you spend a lot of time staring at a computer, you may already need additional support for your eye health. The increased use of computers and video display terminals (VDTs) at home and work has led to an increased need for vision-supporting supplements." [13.]

Whilst I have concentrated on degenerative eye diseases in this book, there are other eye diseases that occur in eyes at any age. The advice given here may help the health of *every* body, including most eye conditions except wet AMD.

It is worth remembering that some people have genetic conditions and injuries that may not improve despite the best nutrition. However, it is always worth the effort to improve your diet because good nutrition helps the body heal and prevents many other diseases common in modern western society.

The advice given in the following chapters is, of necessity, general in nature, and may not apply to all persons. Please be aware that medical research is updating understanding of eye disease all the time. For the latest developments in knowledge regarding your eye disease, it is important to ask your eye doctor.

Three

Things that can Damage your Eyes

Aging

We all age and we cannot press the pause button. It happens. However, you can improve the *quality* of your life, and maybe your eyesight too, as you become older by taking care of the following aspects:

Smoking

Do not smoke tobacco. Smoking has been linked to macular degeneration, and is believed to be linked to cardiovascular disease, which may also affect the eyes and vision.[10.]

Tobacco smoking has the potential to damage your eyesight seriously, as well as the rest of your health. If you are a smoker, you might consider joining a 'Quit' program.

In my late teens, I smoked to allay anxiety. When I grew up, I gave up. I found other methods to deal with anxiety, such as deep relaxation, painting, music, mindfulness, yoga and physical exercise. The latter is the most potent medicine of all.

Sunlight

You need to protect your eyes from direct sunlight. UV rays can penetrate eyelids and directly into your eyes.

Most people know they should never gaze directly at the sun. It can burn the retina of your eyes. However, did you know that because your eyelids are merely a thin layer of skin and membrane, they might cut out some light when we close them, but they do not stop the sun's rays penetrating to your eyeballs? [14]

In Australia, especially in the northern half of the continent, you should protect your eyes if you are out doors in the middle of the day and especially in the hotter months when the midday sun is directly overhead. However, sunlight is good for our skin, stimulating the production of hormones like Vitamin D and melatonin. [15]

There is plenty of evidence to show that Vitamin D supports your mood, your immune system, your bones **and your eyesight**. [Ibid]

Enjoying a sunny day can improve your eyesight and brain function, though staring into direct sunlight is not good for your eyes. Natural outdoor light exposure helps the brain to function brilliantly. *It also stimulates your eyes' photosensitive cells.*

Eyes fail to grow correctly when not exposed to bright outdoor sunlight. Sunlight seems to help children's eyes engage in a healthy cycle. Vision researchers suspect that sunlight triggers a response that aligns distance between the retina and the lens. The eyes are triggered to focus in a way that is not triggered by low indoor lighting.[15, 16.]

Make it a habit to walk or garden in bright sunshine for a minimum of half an hour a day, preferably early in the morning. Being outdoors to gain early morning light on a regular basis is the best way to adjust your ability to go to sleep before midnight. Sunbathing without sunscreen for five minutes on each your back and front before 10.30 am or after 3.30 is very good for your skin and your mental health.

Beware: Some medications require you to stay out of the sun.

Obviously, you need to minimise the amount of time you expose your body, especially if your skin is very pale. It would be best to build up slowly from a minute or two on any exposed area. Even in mid-winter, when the sun is lower in the sky and vitamin D production in the skin is limited, sunlight appears to have health benefits on mood and possibly other beneficial effects.

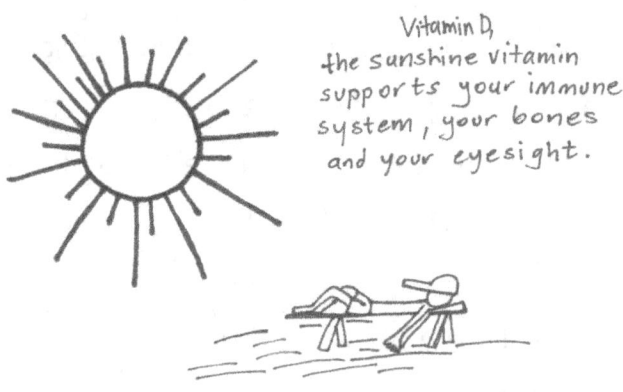

Exposing your skin to the sun can improve your general health and your eyes

Melatonin and vitamin D adjust your sleep/waking cycle. Both of these substances are available as supplements. Six to ten hours sleep is important for the health of all our physical and mental systems, eyesight included. Insufficient sleep may be caused by insufficient melatonin and vitamin D, which interferes with your circadian rhythm. However, with sufficient sunlight early in the day, much of what you need is supplied naturally.[17.]

Glare and Reflected Light

We need to limit our exposure to glare and reflected light.[13.] Screen glare is just one form of reflected light. Most computer screens these days provide an anti-glare function or have a means of turning down the glare. Otherwise, there are protective products that you can buy to place over the screen.

People are using smart mobile phones more and more, as their functions are now those of a mini computer. As a result, people are using their devices outdoors, while waiting for transport, while travelling on public transport and many younger people seem to be seldom without a screen in front of them. It is important to adjust the light on the screen of your phone so that it is not too bright.
Ibid.

When snow skiing or & ice skating, sunlight will reflect glare off the icy ground surface, back onto your face and under the brim of your hat. It will also reflect off the metal frame of your spectacles. This not only endangers your eyesight, but also predisposes you to skin cancers.

Water: swimming, sailing and water skiing provide the same situation where the glare is reflected from the water surface back onto your face and under the brim of your hat. Repeated exposure to glare may promote eye disease.

Wear quality sunglasses.

Obesity

You need to be cautious about what foods you consume. Highly processed foods eaten as a major part of your diet are not good for you. Super-sized foods may soon lead to a super-sized you.[18.]

Eat quality food and nutrients.

Although there are other causes of obesity, if you live on processed and fast food, you may well become obese.

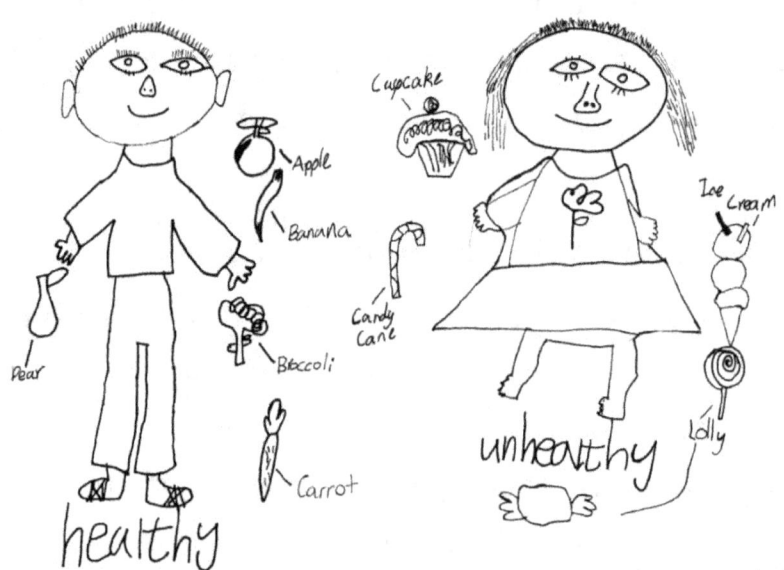

High consumption of fast foods contributes to obesity

Sugar and use of seed oils contribute to inflammation in the body. The consumption of polyunsaturated cooking oils ('vegetable', soy, cottonseed, peanut, canola, corn, sunflower and rice bran oils) are all detrimental, not only to your eyes, but to your entire health.[12, 19] Inflammation is now linked to many diseases, including heart disease and Alzheimer's.[20]

The very worst ingredients for your health are white cane sugar and glucose syrup, vegetable oil and processed white flour.[12, 19]

These oils are very high in inflammatory omega 6 fatty acids (See Ch. 5). Soy, cottonseed and canola oils are also likely to be oxidised and contaminated with remnants of weed killers like glyphosate and the solvents used to remove it.[19, 21]

A healthy body needs only tiny amounts of polyunsaturated oils from fresh nuts and seeds.

Lack of Exercise

"The limited available evidence suggests that regular exercise protects against cataract and age related macular degeneration, two of the leading causes of vision loss in Australia."[22]

Just as our body needs exercise, **our eyes also need exercise.**[21] They rely on muscles and like all muscles, they need exercising too. Our eyes need to move, to change their focal distance frequently.

If you are focusing on a screen or book all day, your eyes will have little time to focus on things that are more distant. If you work in an office on a computer, take a break to stretch every half hour. In addition, while you are stretching your body, stretch your eyes. Look about the room, up at the corners of the ceiling, down at the floor and out of the window. Gaze at things near and far.[23.]

Exercise is also important to keep your blood circulating efficiently.

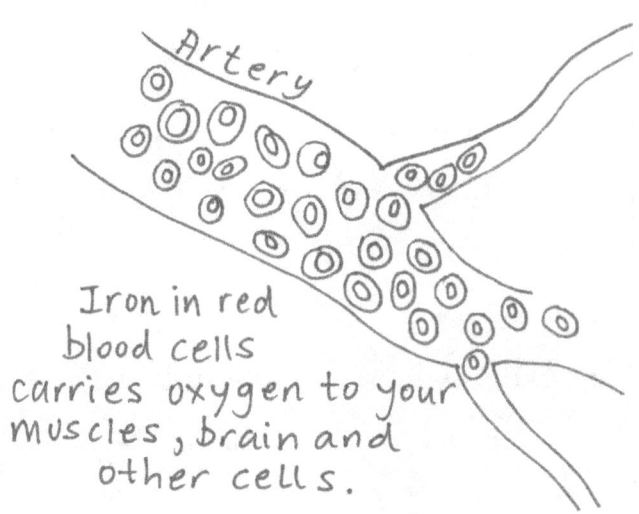

When we exercise, our blood takes oxygen and other nutrients around our body, including to our eyes

When your blood circulation is poor, the nutrients in your food do not circulate to where they are needed in your brain and to your eyes.[22.]

Use the stairs instead of the lift. Walk up and down the escalator. Park two or three blocks from the station and walk to your stop. Garden and play outdoors with your grandchildren.

High and Low Blood Pressure

When blood pressure is too low or too high, it has an effect on the eyes. [18.] When patients are too aggressively treated for their high blood pressure, it can possibly hurt the eye. Certain blood pressure pills have been linked to worsening glaucoma. Both diuretics and calcium channel blockers have a strong link with the progression of glaucoma, according to Laurie Barber.

Ask your doctor for medicine that will not harm your eyesight. The ACE inhibitors appear to have no visual contraindications.[24.] No matter what healthy actions you take, you cannot stop aging.

Even if you eat well, exercise regularly, avoid glare, cigarette smoke and drugs of all kinds, you will probably develop cataracts and maybe some other eye problem. You can do only so much about your genetic inheritance.

It is wise to see an optician to have your eyes tested regularly, especially if you find yourself squinting.

If there are no problems revealed, take advice as to when you should have another test.

In Australia, Medicare covers basic tests so it won't cost you anything if there's nothing wrong. Everyone – not just adults, but kids too – should have their eyes tested periodically.

If there is something wrong with your eyes, it is better to have it treated early than allow the problem to become serious.

Inflammation

Low grade, chronic inflammation is an indication that there is something seriously wrong in our bodies. Inflammation often starts in the mouth.[25] Some very interesting on-going research has revealed that a fourth kind of micro-organism called **archaea** is the culprit. When this organism was first found in deep undersea vents three decades ago, it was thought to be an anaerobic bacterium. Now, we know it is an ancient microbe that pre-dates bacteria, viruses and fungi and has some features which clearly distinguish it from bacteria.

Archaea are found in volcanic vents on land too, and in sulphur laden water. More recently, they have been found in animal guts, including in humans, and in particular, in our mouths. Like the other, better-known micro-organisms, there are numerous kinds of archaea. Much more needs to be discovered about how these organisms are related to degenerative diseases like macular degeneration and heart disease.[25, 26, 27]

Medications and their Side Effects

It is always important to know the side effects of all medications you take. This applies to both prescribed and over the counter medications.[24, 28, 29, 30]

Be cautious about whatever you put into your mouth and onto your skin. Make sure you know it is safe.

Nearly all medications have side effects. This includes herbal medicines. Some of those side effects might affect your vision.

> "Many different medications can cause eye problems," says Laurie Barber, MD, a spokeswoman for the American Academy of Ophthalmology. "Some of these side effects are minor, like dryness. Others are more serious."[24]

Medications like diuretics, antihistamines, antidepressants, cholesterol-lowering drugs, beta-blockers and birth control pills can cause Dry Eye.

"... common systemic medications that cause ocular side effects include: bisphosphonates; cyclosporine and tacrolimus; minocycline; hydroxychloroquine; ethambutol; topiramate; tamsulosin; amiodarone; anticholinergics; erectile dysfunction drugs; blood pressure medications; and some herbal medications." [30.]

Herbal Medications and Nutritional Supplements

The sale of nutritional and herbal medications is a multi-billion dollar industry worldwide.

"Basically half of the population takes some sort of nutritional supplement or herbal medicine, and half of those people don't tell their doctors about it because they don't think it's pertinent," says Dr. Fraunfelder. "However, it can be pertinent, because sometimes herbal medications can interact with prescription medicines the patient is already taking. For instance, ginkgo biloba causes patients to have a longer bleeding time, so it can make people who take blood thinners more prone to bleeding." [30.]

As I found from my own experience, it is inadvisable to **spend time in bright sunshine if you are taking St John's Wort for anxiety.** I was reading outside and soon, both my eyes became very inflamed and felt gritty. The inflammation disappeared a few days after I stopped taking St. John's Wort.

The herbal medicine **Glycyrrhiza glabra or liquorice is a perennial herb of the pea family (Fabaceae).**

> **Fraunfelder** says "...black bitter *licorice has side effects on the eyes* and may also cause migraine headaches with visual side effects." [Ibid.]

Canthaxanthin, which can be taken orally as a tanning agent and is used in some foods as a colouring agent, can deposit small crystals in the retina of the eye.[30.]

Canthaxanthin is a natural antioxidant found in some, but not all, wild mushrooms and, in that natural state, it is helpful for our eyes. The chemical used for tanning is synthetic. [30.]

Synthetic Chemicals

Some chemicals produced in laboratories are close to nature identical and some are mirror images. The main reasons why industry doesn't make nature identical chemicals is usually to do with the company's ability to patent the product. (See p. 61

for more about 'handedness' of synthetic molecules.')

Many synthetic chemicals are counter-productive to our health, although their natural form is beneficial.

Ask Your Pharmacist or Prescribing Doctor

Your pharmacist or doctors are the best people to ask about interactions between drugs and supplements. If you have problems with your eyes, always ask if the drug being prescribed could interfere with your eyes by itself or by interaction with something else you are taking. There may be a suitable alternative.

Supplements can also have unwanted side effects under some circumstances. Check with your eye doctor that what you are intending to take is safe for you. Always tell your doctor if you are taking ginko biloba, vitamin E and fish oils, especially if you intend to have surgery. These are natural blood thinners.

Four

Foods that can Damage your Eyes

Problems with eyesight can strike us at any age, but more of us seem to have difficulties as we age. Now that many of us live well into our eighties or nineties, problems with cataracts are a particular province of older people, but so are glaucoma, macular degeneration, dry eye and diabetic retinopathy.

Say "No" to processed 'foods' such as cereals, biscuits, cakes, prepared meals and sauces. They are full of sugars, glucose syrups typically from wheat and corn, polyunsaturated oils, refined flour, soy, preservatives, synthetic antioxidants and colourings. If these processed foods form a major part of your diet, you might expect obesity, chronic ill health and degenerative eye disease.[12, 19, 32, 33]

Sugar

There are many types of sugar in processed foods. The letters 'ose' on the end of the name indicates it is a sugar: sucrose, glucose, dextrose, maltose, fructose etc.

Highly refined sugar from sugar cane, sugar beet and corn (maize) are all stripped of minerals and other nutrients during processing. These nutrients are required for the proper digestion of sugar. Consequently, the zinc, chromium, copper, calcium, vitamin B6 and other nutrients needed for proper digestion are drawn from your blood and bone reserves, depleting your body of these necessary vitamins and minerals.[12, 32.]

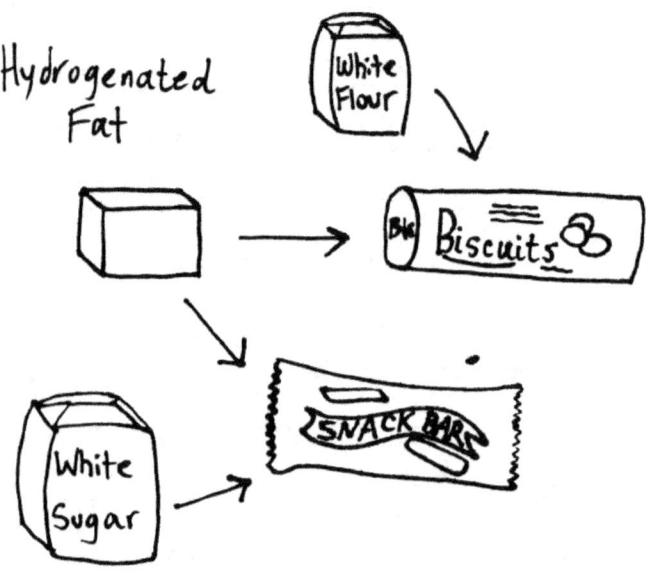

Processed foods lead to inflammation and disease

Worse, even a moderate, regular intake of sugar may interfere with insulin production and other bodily processes, ultimately leading to diabetes and cardiovascular disease, the two biggest killers in the western world; both are linked to eye disease.

Note also the link with sugar to diabetic retinopathy.

This is why nutritionists call refined white sugar 'white death'.[12.]

Starch

Refined grains like white flour, white rice and pasta from wheat or corn, readily break down into sugar (glucose) and increase inflammation.[12.]

Highly processed flours from wheat, or whatever grain, affect our bodies in much the same way as sugars. The nutrients (e.g. zinc and vitamin E) from the bran and germ of the grain are stripped off, leaving behind pure starch. Once again, the body draws on our reserves of nutrients to digest these non-foods, depleting our muscles and bones.

Starch is readily converted into sugar (glucose) and so the damage it does is the same as sucrose and the other sugars hidden in processed foods. [Ibid]

Soy

There is much research showing that soy may be helpful in menopause because it contains chemicals called isoflavones that mimic oestrogen. This research was initiated because, when the Americans occupied Japan after WWII, they noticed that Japanese women did not suffer from the same menopausal symptoms as American women. Asians eat *fermented* soy that they make into foods and sauces such as tofu, tempeh and miso. The fermentation process is the key to making soy healthy. Unfermented soy products are not so good for us.[12]

Unfortunately, in the USA, they turned their huge soybean crops into soy oil, soy flour and soymilk.

Fats and Oils

The body can make most of the types of fatty acids we require. However, some we cannot make. These are called **essential fatty acids.** They **must** come from our food or supplements.

The major essential fatty acids are called omega 3 and omega 6. They are found in polyunsaturated oils, including fish oils [19]

Most polyunsaturated oils in the supermarket come from seeds. Industrial seed oils are made from soybeans, sunflower seeds, canola seed, safflower seed, corn and cottonseeds. Peanuts are a legume, but peanut oil is also a mass-produced vegetable oil. Those labelled 'vegetable oil' are blended from whatever is cheapest on the market - often cotton seed oil - which contains remnants of weed killers like glyphosate, and peanut oil, which may contain aflatoxin residue. Aflatoxin is a fungus that targets peanuts and can cause allergies [23, 34].

These seed oils are cheap, and are usually sold in one or two litre plastic bottles that have no protection against light. The oils are processed using petro chemical solvents like hexane, tiny remnants of which remain in the oils. Also, the plastic bottle sheds tiny fragments of plastic and any oils stored in them may absorb this micro plastic.[33, 34] In turn, your body will absorb the remnants of disease-producing micro plastics, herbicide and pesticide chemicals.

Some omega 6 fatty acids are essential in our diet. These are best obtained from grains, vegetables, fresh nuts and two fruits, avocado and olives.

The ratio of Omega 6 to omega 3 fatty acids in our diets is incredibly important. The problem comes when we consume too much omega 6.

We need to keep our omega 6 levels no more than six times the omega 3 ratio. That is an absolute maximum. The closer the ratio is to 1:1, the better for our health.[12, 19]

Why do we need these two types of fatty acids to be in a close ratio?

Excess Omega 6 fats promote inflammation; omega 3 fats fight inflammation.

Over the thousands of years that human beings were hunters and gatherers, they lived by rivers, lakes and the seaside. The women gathered shellfish as a staple part of the family diet. I saw this in 2006 in New Caledonia, where the village women still scour the reef every low tide for edible seafood. Witness also the Aboriginal shell middens that they see as an indicator of residence in traditional times. Before agriculture was established over the past two plus thousand years ago, shellfish formed the staple diet along with small animals. People supplemented these foods with roots, nuts, seeds and berries. The fish and animals all provided an ideal ratio of omega 3:6 essential fatty acids. Omega three is sadly missing from the modern western diet.

If you do not counter the highly inflammatory seed oils in your diet with omega 3 oils and fats, you may become prone to all sorts of disease, including dementia and eye disease.

Inflammation and disease tend to go together.

Inflammation is involved in all modern western diseases that are chronic: cardiovascular disease, diabetes, eye disease, obesity, high blood pressure, kidney disease, Alzheimer's, cancer etc.[19.]

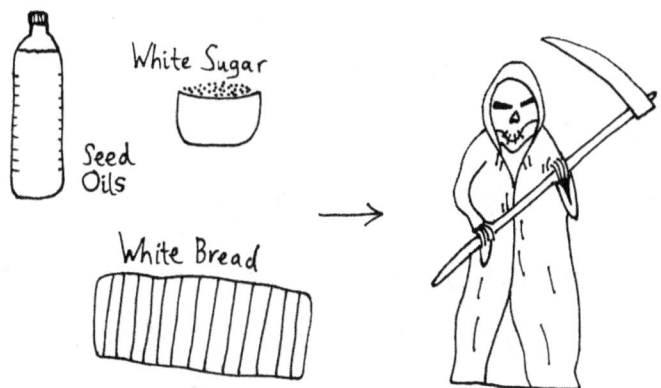

Seed oils, refined sugars and wheat together create inflammation, degenerative diseases and early death

Some people take fish oil supplements and eat *wild*, cold-water, fatty fish like mackerel, sardines and salmon because these fish have high levels of anti-inflammatory omega 3 fats. In the wild, salmon eat algae that contain the precursors for omega 3 fatty acids. [Ibid.] Tuna is lower in EFAs.

Farmed salmon is available frozen in Australian supermarkets. In Tasmania, Australia, *Tassal* and *Huon* fish farms produce salmon. They list the foods they feed to their fish, but, can farmed salmon access algae? We need to keep note of the diet fed to farmed salmon. Make sure you read the fine print with a magnifying glass to check the country of origin and the amounts of DHA and EPA, which are the specific chemicals we need in omega 3 fatty acids. Some northern European fish farmers reportedly add canola oil to the diets of their growing fish. If this is true, it is not good for the essential fatty acid balance in the fish.

Which fats contain more Omega 3?

Mainly fish oils are very high in omega 3 that is bioavailable. Animal fats also contain some omega 3, as do some seed oils. Research suggests little, if any, *plant*-based omega 3 oils are able to be utilised by the human body.[12, 19, 33]

Flaxseed oil has 58 % omega 3 and only 14 % omega 6. **Hemp** has a balance of 20% omega 3 and 60% omega 6. However, these two oils are less bioavailable than salmon or krill oil.[19] At the time of writing hemp oil is easily available only in capsules in Australia.

Most other seed oils have very little, if any, omega 3. Sunflower oil is 75% omega 6. It is frequently used in margarine, making that a very inflammatory product.[19] Manufacturers of margarine and mayonnaise frequently use canola oil. Canola contains only 30% omega 6, but much less omega 3 – only 7%. [Ibid.]

Animal fats

Animal fats like butter, dripping, lard, and also organic coconut oil and palm oil are saturated fats. They are solid at room temperature and **these are the safest fats to use for cooking because they have a higher smoke point.** [Ibid.]

Domestic animal flesh contains more fat than their wild counterparts do. Depending on the diet consumed by the animal, its fat may also contain fewer essential fatty acids. Farmed beef (grass-fed) contains a small percentage of omega 3 fatty acids and no omega 6. By contrast, pork fat contains 10% omega 6 fatty acids and almost no omega 3. [Ibid.] Chicken farming is more intensive and the type of fatty acids in chicken fat is highly dependent on their diet, according to research by Alagawany and others.[35] I believe the diet of the animal is crucial.

Lamb has been dubbed 'land salmon' by Janet McNally because of its fatty acid profile.[38]

> McNally says, "The table shows that lamb — all lamb — indeed has the healthiest omega-6:3

ratio of all the listed land species. Domestic lamb, which was likely raised on pasture but finished on grain, has a healthier ratio than beef, with significantly higher omega-3 content compared to both conventional and grass-fed beef."

Figure 3: Essential fatty acid content in land animals

Per 170 grams or 6 oz. serving	% fat	Omega 6	Omega 3	Ratio 6/3
Pork ground. raw	21	2830 mg	119 mg	23.8 1
Chicken ground. raw	8	2229	162	13.8 1
Beef ground. raw	21	732	80	9.15 1
Grassfed beef ground. raw	14	720	148	4.87 1
Domestic lamb raw composite (1)	19	1851	560	3.3 1
Domestic lamb shoulder steak (2)	19	1918	543	3.5 1
NZ lamb. raw composite (1)	17	713	526	1.35 1
US grassfed lamb experiment. raw*	20	1654	2147	0.77 1
Farmed Atlantic salmon. raw	14	1746	4455	0.39 1
Wild Atlantic salmon. raw	6.5	292	3588	0.08 1

*Composite of shoulder and sirloin steaks from 10 lambs. Lambs were fed a pasture mix that included kale. tilage radish. ryegrass. hairy vetch. and red clover.
(1) composite of retail cuts trimmed to 1 8 inch fat
(2) shoulder blade steak trimmed to 1 8 inch fat

Of land animals, lamb has the healthiest ratio of omega 3 and omega 6.
Table copied from article by Janet McNally.

McNally says, "The New Zealand lamb, which I assume was finished on forages [grasses], has less omega-6 fatty acid compared to domestic [USA] lamb and a more desirable fatty acid ratio. But none of these meats were really comparable to salmon in total omega-3 content and omega-6:3 ratio." Ibid.

Hydrogenated fats

Hydrogenated fats, just like animal fats, are solid at room temperature, but as a result of processing.

The process of hydrogenating fats creates disease-producing trans-fatty acids.

Trans-fatty acids are widely thought to cause cancers and they damage our eyesight. It is also important not to burn fats.

Burning any fats and oils until they smoke causes the production of cancer-causing acrylamide as well as trans-fatty acids.[19.]

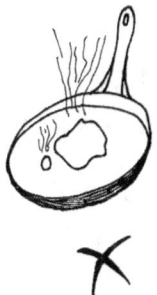

Rancid Foods

Rancid foods taste and smell bitter.

The main cause of rancidity of fats is oxidation caused by exposure to heat, light and air.

Lite Oils' – have been extra bleached. One gram of oil or fat is always equivalent to nine calories or close to 38 kilojoules.[19]

Mono-saturated oils

Mono-saturated oils, like virgin olive oil, hemp, linseed, avocado and walnut oil, are excellent to use on salads. Keep such oils in a cool dark cupboard in a well-stoppered glass bottle.

These oil contains little in the way of essential fatty acids, but they have other important health benefits. (see Table 2. p. 47).

> According to the website for macular degeneration, "...recent research shows those who consume one tablespoon of olive oil per day are less likely to develop late stage age-related macular degeneration. More research is required into this area."[39]

Polyunsaturated oils

Most polyunsaturated oils oxidise much more quickly than mono-saturated oils and saturated fats.

All whole grains, nuts and seeds as well as the oils made from them need to be kept away from *heat*, *light and air.*[19.] They should be kept in dark coloured glass jars or bottles, firmly capped and stored in a cool dark cupboard (or in the fridge during very hot conditions).

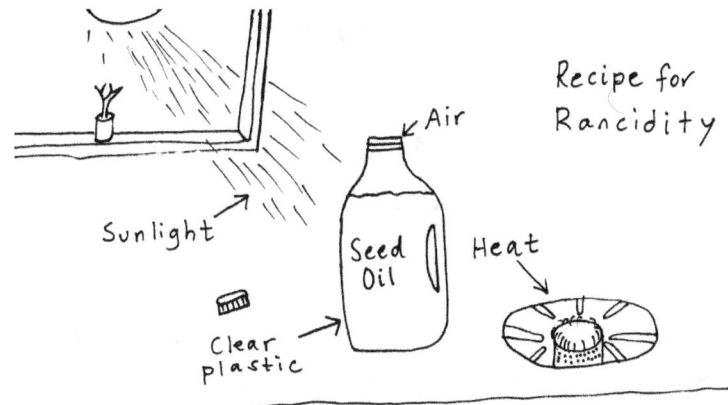

Light, air and heat oxidise oils and fats, turning then rancid

If you must use a vegetable oil, never leave the bottle next to the stove. That is a recipe for producing rancidity, also known as oxidation. [Ibid.]

Dr Chris Knobbe, an ophthalmologist in the USA has been on a crusade since 2015 to teach us about the toxicity of vegetable oils.[25.] He says, *"...vegetable oil seeds are crushed, heated, pressed. They go through about four or five heatings ... then they go to a petroleum drive, hexane solvent bath, And then they're steamed, degummed ... they go through a chemical process of being alkalinized (sic), bleached and deodorized before they go into this bottle and we think they're healthy. They're extraordinarily oxidized. They're toxic."*

Air (oxygen), light and heat destroy unsaturated oils by quickly turning them rancid. Avoid them as much as possible.

Fresh nuts and seeds, olives and avocados are the best source of polyunsaturated oils – natural and unheated so that they are not oxidised.

The Microbial Connection

The connection between high omega 6 essential fatty acids and *archaea* has not yet been fully explored. Both contribute to inflammatory disease.

The archaea microbe, mentioned in chapter 3 (pp 33-35) continues to be intensely researched. What is known is that when the microbial organisms in our bodies are out of balance, they give an advantage to one kind over another which allows disease to enter. Where that disease will attack is due to a combination of environmental factors and genetic weaknesses.[27.] The role of this recently discovered microbe in the inflammatory process is still in its infancy. In the meantime, *cutting back severely on your intake of polyunsaturated oils and sugars are an excellent way to take control of the disease process in your body.*

Five

More about Fats and Oils

General knowledge in the community about the chemistry of fats and oils is limited. The topic has been the centre of false advertising and much misinformation, even within the medical field. I shall do my best to simplify the facts without misconstruing them.

This chapter deals in more detail with the chemistry of oils. If you want to, skip ahead to chapter six.

The large and chemically detailed textbook by Udo Erasmus, *Fats that Heal and Fats that Kill*, is the source of most of my information regarding fats and oils. It is an enormously helpful resource. (See reference 20.)

Fat is an essential part of a healthy diet. About one third of a healthy body consists of fat.

A gram of fat contains about three times the energy of a gram of carbohydrate or protein (nine calories). About one third of our energy intake (in calories or kilojoules, not grams) should be in fat. That means you need to consume about 70 – 100 grams of fat in your food each day to repair and renew the healthy fats in your body.[19.] The total kilojoules you require will depend on both body size *and* the level of energy you expend.

Our entire nervous system and brains are encased in fats and our hormones are made from cholesterol, a type of fat. Fat also acts as a shock absorber to protect our internal organs such as our kidneys, liver and heart. Body fat is the body's way of conserving energy for times of food shortage or famine.

Females have a little more fat under their skin to make their bodies softer and to conserve energy in case of pregnancy. It is also nature's way of making them more attractive to the opposite sex.

Our brains and nervous systems require essential fatty acids from our diet to maintain health. Consuming too much of the wrong kinds of fats and oils leads to inflammation and degenerative disease, including eye disease, diabetes and dementia.

We need to eat the parts of an animal that contain the nutrients we require to keep our own body parts repaired. This is the reason hunter-gatherer people ate the heart, liver and other organs of the animals they hunted. Lamb brains, for example, are a high source of essential fatty acids and zinc. Lamb itself has plenty of omega 3 and omega 6 fatty acids.[39.]

The ideal diet would contain omega 3 and omega 6 fatty acids in a ratio of 1:1.

Currently in the USA, **people consume more than 25 times as much inflammatory omega 6 oils as they do non-inflammatory oils**. These seed oils are found in nearly all processed foods and a lot of café and restaurant foods as well.[19.] Australians follow closely on the heels of the USA in consumption of processed and restaurant foods.

The industrial seed oil industry barely existed before the Second World War. It was a fledgling industry around the beginning of the twentieth century. After WW II, the US government encouraged the growing of more seed crops for oils.

Over the next three decades, with the help of companies like multi-national Monsanto that took control of seed genetics, these crops and their oils spread throughout the world.[12.]

In February 1999, there were riots in Indonesia because the price of cooking oil and rice soared. This happened again in 2008 and several times since. In Bangladesh among the middle classes, as in Indonesia, seed oils are favoured over the much healthier palm oil for cooking, and there, increasing numbers of people suffer from obesity, cardiovascular disease and diabetes. These diseases were rare in SE Asia when palm and coconut oils were the main source of fats pre WWII.* (See p. 56.)

Diabetes, cardiovascular disease and cancer have become huge health problems in SE Asia as well as in the USA and Australia now that seed oils are the staple fat consumed. Degenerative diseases were almost unknown 120 years ago in the USA, at the turn of last century. Most optometrists rarely saw macular degeneration before 1920, and then only rarely. ^{Ibid.}

Cottonseed is used for animal food, which alters the essential fatty acid balance of animal fat. In addition, oil is extracted from the seeds for human consumption. Nowadays, cotton is mostly a genetically modified crop and tiny remnants of glyphosate weed killer remain in the oil after processing. In Australia, most canola is also

'*Roundup* ready'. *Roundup* is the brand name for the weed killer, glyphosate.[23.]

There is considerable evidence linking glyphosate application to crops and non-Hodgkin's cancer, although the evidence is controversial. It is, at the time of writing, being fought in the courts in the USA and a class action is about to commence in Australia.[41.]

Plastic bottles shed tiny fragments of plastic and any oils stored in them may absorb chemicals from the plastic.[33.]

Saturated Oils and Fats

A saturated fat is one where the chain of fatty acids has no free spaces for a free radical electron from oxygen to pair with an electron on a carbon molecule.

A whole lot of light and heat is needed to break the bonds of the carbon and hydrogen molecules so that an oxygen electron can pair with the carbon instead. This makes **saturated fats the most stable of all fats.**[19.] (See the diagram on p.55.)

Saturated fats are solid at room temperature. Examples of saturated fats used for food are from animal products (dripping and lard, butter and cream) and from coconut and palm oils. Most saturated fats contain very little essential fatty acids, though they do contain other nutritionally important fatty acids that we should not disregard. Meat and fats from beasts on organic pasture are best.

Mono-saturated oils

Mono-saturated oils are liquid at room temperature. They have one free space for an electron from an oxygen molecule to pair up with the carbon molecules in the fatty acid chain. This makes them not quite as stable as saturated fats. These oils contain several important fatty acids for our diets, though little in the way of omega 3 or 6. See table on page 38.

Olive oil, and some tree nut oils like macadamia, almond and walnut are mono-saturated oils. Avocados are also high in mono-saturated fats. Like sesame oil, the oils from olives, avocados and almonds contain their own natural antioxidants. [Ibid.] If you intend to use these oils on your food, buy them in small quantities. They should be virgin first-pressing oils that will still go off more quickly than saturated fats. It has been claimed that some of the olive oils sourced from southern Europe have been found to be adulterated with cheaper oils. Australia and New Zealand produce their own high quality virgin olive and avocado oils.

Polyunsaturated Oils

Polyunsaturated oils are the most unstable of all. They have many spaces in their chains of fatty acids where a free oxygen molecule can pair up with a carbon molecule. The most widely available are the seed and legume oils discussed in chapter 4. Being mass-produced, seed oils are cheap to buy, but toxic to consume.[25] It is healthier to eat fresh nuts, seeds, olives and avocados.

Polyunsaturated oils contain high quantities of omega 6 fatty acids. We require some of these fatty acids, but nowhere near the amount found in modern processed foods.

Fish Oils

Most omega 3 oils come from the sea. The rhyming of three and sea helps us remember which essential fatty acid is which.

If you decide to take fish oil supplements to counter the omega 6 in your food, be careful of the source of the supplement. Cheap, oil based supplements are more likely to be rancid already and many contain heavy metals.

Only buy reputable brands of oil from wild salmon and krill or, better still, consume several servings of very fresh, frozen or canned wild fish each week. Salmon, mackerel, sardines and herring are the best sources. There is some omega 3 in tuna, but not nearly as much as advertisers would have you believe. There's more in grass-fed lamb.

Krill oil is perhaps the best source of omega 3 oils as a supplement, as these tiny crustaceans are harvested from the icy waters of the Southern Ocean where pollution levels are still very low. However, krill is one tiny species of many that make up plankton – the food at the very bottom of the food chain. All animals rely on this basic foundation for food. Human beings are not noted for adopting sustainable fishing habits until the product is severely threatened. Thus, I am wary of recommending a product that is often sourced unsustainably.

It is not simple. Most essential fatty acids are in polyunsaturated oils or wild fish. Not all seed oils are bad for you. Small amounts of high quality polyunsaturated fats are good for you – just not too much, and they must be in balance with omega3.

Omega 3 fatty acids have their precursors in marine algae. Fish that eat the algae convert the fats into omega 3 which humans are then able to digest.

Figure 2: Oils and Fats – type of Fat content

Type of Lipid	Saturated	Mono-saturated	Poly-unsaturated Omega 3	Poly-unsaturated Omega 6	Other
Beef Dripping	46	39	1	3	12
Butter	51	24	1	2	21
Canola oil	7	59	9	20	5
Chicken fat	27	41	1	18	14
Coconut oil	84	6	0	1	9
Corn oil	12	24	1	56	7
Cottonseed oil	25	17	0	50	8
Hemp oil	9	11	21	59	0
Lard (pig fat)	36	41	1	9	13
Olive oil X virgin	13	71	1	8	7
Palm oil	48	36	0	9	8
Peanut oil	16	44	0	31	9
Rice bran oil	25	38	2	32	3
Sesame oil	14	39	0	40	8
Soy oil	14	23	6	49	7
Sunflower oil	10	19	0	64	7

1. The amounts are shown in grams / 100 grams.
2. I used data from https:www.skillsyouneed.com/ps/fats-oils.html to create this table.

As you can see from the table, hemp oil is one of the best-balanced products. However, only a small percentage of humans are able to convert omega 3 into DHA and EPA the crucial chemicals humans require from omega 3. If hemp could convert omega 3 to DHA and EPA, it would be perfect for all humans and solve a problem for vegans![39.] Vegetable omega 3s do contain a third *essential* fatty acid though – ALA (alpha linolenic acid). Details about the importance of ALA are only just emerging.

Rancidity

Oxidation can cause rancidity and the development of **trans-fatty acids.** This can happen when lipids (oils and fats) are exposed to **heat**, light and oxygen, during microwave cooking, and frying. All oils and fats can overheat during frying. Add water first. If the oil smokes or burns, discard it.[19.]

Margarines and Hydrogenation

The margarine manufacturing industry uses seed oils, hydrogenation and antioxidants to produce their products. Hydrogenation is a process that forces hydrogen molecules into the fatty acid chains under **heat** and pressure to make them solid at room temperature. Manufacturers of margarines hydrogenise their product enough to make it soft and spreadable at room temperature and most use synthetic antioxidants to protect the fats.[19, 42, 43] Hydrogenation is the process that frequently causes trans-fats[20] and oxidation.[25]

Trans-fats

Trans-fats are created when the heat and pressure applied in hydrogenation twists the chemical bonds of the molecules. These fats become solid at room temperature and such twisted fats are dangerous to our health.[12, 19, 42, 43] They become carcinogenic (cancer causing) and governments have introduced legislation limiting the percentage of trans-fats permitted in our foodstuffs.

It is also possible to create trans-fats in microwave ovens. Microwaves do not heat food evenly. They can overheat small portions of the food to the extent that fat molecules can twist into trans-fats.[19]

It is not advisable to cook foods that contain fat in a microwave.

Oxidation

When iron *oxidises*, it rusts. Without protection, shiny iron soon takes on a reddish patina of rust, a powdery substance. Similarly, when aluminium oxidises, it develops a powdery coating of grey 'rust'.

Not just minerals rust. Inside the human body, lipids (i.e. fats and oils) also oxidise or rust.

Mass produced seed oils are heated until they become oxidised and rancid. Then they are deodorized so the consumer doesn't notice.

Oxidative rancidity is "a chemical reaction catalysed by heat, ultraviolet light, heavy metals and oxygen." [19, 32, 42]

Oxidation takes place when the carbon molecular chain has spaces for not only hydrogen atoms, but also free radical electrons from oxygen molecules. This process proceeds by a free radical chain reaction mechanism.[19] Free radical oxygen molecules will pair themselves with carbon molecules in chains of fatty acids, producing oxidation that is linked to inflammation.

Foods can deteriorate by oxidation both outside and inside our bodies. Oxidation has more effects on lipids (oils and fats) than carbohydrates. Lipid peroxidation is where "... free radicals 'steal' electrons from the lipids in cell membranes, resulting in cell damage." [19]

Figure 3: Unpaired electrons become free radicals

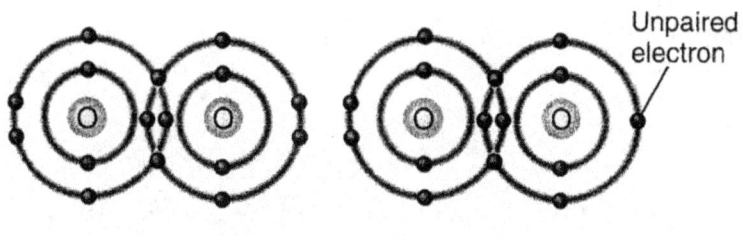

(a) Oxygen molecule   (b) Superoxide free radical

A free radical has an unpaired electron in its outer shell

Source: Tortora and Grabowski, (1996).
"Principles of Anatomy and Physiology", p 87.

Cell membranes are made of phospholipids – a chemical constructed of both fat and phosphorus. If the lipid part of the molecule is damaged, we become ill. It is essential to maintain the integrity of the cell wall.

Inside the cell, we have mitochondria, sometimes hundreds of them. They also require integrity in their walls, which also contain lipids. Mitochondria provide our energy.

Processed foods can lead to degenerative eye disease and other health problems

Oxidised fats and oils are a serious contributor to all major eye diseases.

Antioxidants are the chemicals that derail the process of oxidation. You will learn about these chemicals in the next chapter.

* Re Palm oil: Whilst palm oil is a healthy dietary fat, the cutting down of rainforest habitat for orangutans and other native animals to supply the world with this product is unsustainable.

Six
Antioxidants to the rescue

The body uses antioxidants from foods and supplements to counter the immense harm caused by oxidation (the breakdown of an oxygen molecule).

Natural antioxidants are vitamins A, C, E, Zinc, carotenes (beta-carotene, lutein, zeaxanthin, astaxanthin) and anthocyanins.[32, 46, 47, 48, 49]

These antioxidants are extremely important in maintaining not just general health, but also eye health.

Manufacturers of processed foods add synthetic antioxidants to their products to increase their shelf life. Some synthetic antioxidants are nature identical, some are mirror image chemicals and some are tweaked so that they can be patented. Synthetic antioxidants may be harmful inside the body.[33, 49, 51]

You can check for additive codes in a book like The *Additive Code Breaker* or on the internet.[52] Antioxidant additives have additive codes in the 300s. Natural antioxidants extracted from plants are numbered from 300 to 306. Those numbered from 307 to 321 are laboratory-sourced antioxidants, which may have side effects. The identification numbers are printed on the labels of manufactured foods. (Note: in Europe, additive numbers have an E in front e.g. E300.)

Manufacturers tend to list ingredients in very small print. That makes me wonder if they are trying to hide something. If you cannot read the ingredients, maybe you could follow my lead and refuse to buy the product. You could photograph the label on your smart phone and then enlarge the picture or, as a last resort, carry a small magnifying glass. The more ingredient numbers the worse the food is likely to be for your health.

Antioxidants and your Eyes

Your eyes are an extension of your brain tissue. The brain and its nerves are made up largely of fats.

Eye problems like macular degeneration, where drusen deposits form in front of your vision, need help from high quality natural antioxidants, which may help slow the deterioration of the eyes.

Unfortunately, to date, no research shows a medical cure for AMD. However, recent research shows a parallel increase in the incidence of age-related macular degeneration since the development of the processed food industry started in the mid-1930s.[12, 19, 25, 51] During the 19th century and very early 20th century, diabetes, heart failure and AMD were rare.[12]

If you eat large amounts of processed foods containing sugars and seed oils, you might expect to develop serious eye diseases and could eventually lose much of your vision.

Antioxidants: Natural vs Synthetic

Natural Antioxidants are protective of eyes. Synthetic antioxidants that are not nature identical may be harmful to people.

Food manufacturers use mostly synthetic antioxidants to protect processed foods from oxidation.[19, 34, 47] Many of these synthetic antioxidants have been shown to be linked to serious side effects in susceptible people, especially those with autoimmune disorders. [26, 28, 51, 53]

The European Union has banned the use of some antioxidants, including DPA (diphenylamine) and ethoxyquin, which are used in the fruit sector in some southern EU countries where they experience high solar irradiation during the fruit production season. [12]

Another group of antioxidants are most commonly used in bread making to prevent the growth of moulds. In particular, the antioxidants 319 – 321 are banned in the European Union, but used in Australia, especially in tropical regions of high humidity like Darwin in the wet season.[12, 53] My husband is very intolerant of this antioxidant.

We need to consume foods and nutrients containing naturally occurring food antioxidants that will do the same job of preventing oxidation inside our bodies.

Oxidation eventually results in degenerative diseases, premature aging and in some cases, cancer. It is especially bad for our eyes.

Vitamins A, C and E are the best-known antioxidants, but there are many others that are particularly good for your eyes, including zinc, astaxanthin, anthocyanins, canthaxanthin, lutein and zeaxanthin.[34, 46, 47, 48, 49, 50]

Vitamin E

Frequently Vitamin E is extracted from wheat germ. If you consume fresh wheat germ, you should keep it in the fridge in an airtight glass jar.

If it smells or tastes bitter, it has gone rancid (oxidised) and should not be consumed.

Look for **d alpha tocopherol** in small letters on the label of a Vitamin E supplement. This is the natural form of vitamin E that your cells can absorb.[12, 18]

Many supplements use _dl alpha tocopherol_. The little 'l' makes all the difference. It stands for left. Chemicals have left and right-handed versions. In the case of vitamin E, only the right-hand version fits the receptors on the cell wall. Its mirror image does not.[19]

Dr Michael Lelah, a research chemist, says, "Unlike other vitamins, synthetic Vitamin E is not biochemically equivalent to the natural forms. Synthetic Vitamin E is a mixture of 8 stereoisomers, only one of which is equivalent to d-alpha-tocopherol. Synthetic Vitamin E is produced from petro-chemicals – by the reaction of isophytpol with trimethylhydrquinone."[51]

Figure 4: Chemical molecules belong to either left or right handed forms

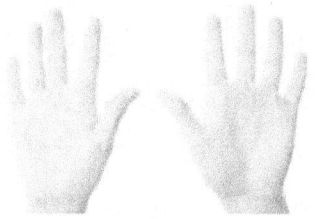

The left-hand synthetic molecule does not fit into the cell receptor

When the left-hand synthetic molecule does not fit into the cell receptor, this is often described as being like trying to put the wrong shaped key in a lock. If the Vitamin E cannot enter the cell, then it cannot do its job. It is just the same as if you tried to open your front door with your key upside down.

Figure 6. Cell binding sites are often compared to keys and keyholes

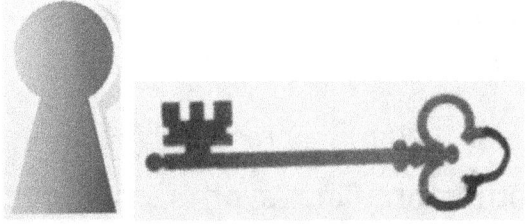

An upside-down key will not fit into the keyhole.

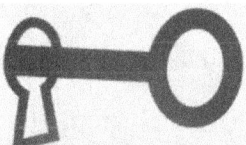

Only the correctly shaped key fits into the keyhole

Millar et al, using Medline and Cochrane metadata, conducted a large data search about the effectiveness of vitamin E as an antioxidant.[56.]

The analysis found that more people died when administered Vitamin E than those who didn't. However, most of the patients in the multiple studies were already suffering from heart disease and other morbidities.

"We searched for all reports of clinical trials (with no language restrictions) that tested the effect of vitamin E supplementation in humans. We performed a MEDLINE search by using ...terms **vitamin E, antioxidant vitamins, alpha tocopherol, tocopherol, and clinical trials**. [My emphasis.] The search period was 1966 through August 2004. We complemented the MEDLINE search by searching the Cochrane database of randomized, controlled trials; reviewing the reference lists from original research, review articles, and previous meta-analyses; and reviewing the files of the investigators ...

'High doses of vitamin E may displace other fat-soluble antioxidants (for example, **γ-tocopherol**), disrupting the natural balance of antioxidant systems and increasing vulnerability to oxidative damage." [Ibid]

It is difficult to know how seriously to take this research when there is no mention of d alpha tocopherol or another valuable type of vitamin E, gamma tocopherol, being used in these studies. I want to know which tocopherols inhibited co-antioxidants. Does synthetic vitamin E have unwanted side effects? Are researchers who use synthetic vitamin E in their studies the ones that find it is ineffective or even detrimental? I suspect it is, especially if taken in large doses, but we need this to be rigorously researched.

Miller et al mention in the literature that gamma tocopherol might have anti-cancer properties. This antioxidant is found naturally in some nuts. The nutrient is not widely known and there are no supplements of it readily available.[58.]

Too much vitamin E could be detrimental, especially if it is synthetic.

Dr Lelah also says, "Synthetic alpha-tocopherol is only *half* as active in the body as the natural form. In review of comparison studies between natural Vitamin E and synthetic Vitamin E in animals and in humans, natural sourced Vitamin E is at least twice as effective as synthetic Vitamin E based on physiological and pharmacological markers. **There are no good studies comparing the effects of natural Vitamin E vs. synthetic Vitamin E on diseases.** [My emphasis] In addition, other work presented at this conference indicates that many of the components of natural Vitamin E, gamma-tocotrienol, for example, have their own specific physiological benefits." [51.]

Vitamin E can thin the blood, so tell your doctor if you are taking a vitamin E supplement. As with fish oils, it can interfere with blood thinners like Warfarin and be contraindicated before surgery.

Vitamin C.

Most of us think of citrus fruits when we want fresh vitamin C. There are other fruits like kiwi and papaya with higher vitamin C content:

1 moderate sized orange (130g) 70mg vit C

1 cup of fresh blackcurrants 202mg vit C

½ cantaloupe 112mg vit C

1 guava (90g) 165mg vit C

2 kiwi fruit (150g) 150mg vit C

1 cup Papaya 187mg vit C

1 cup strawberries 84.5mg vit C [52.]

Fruits have been grown bigger and bigger since 1990, so we need to approximate the amount of a piece of fruit to a standard 250g cooking cup. One and one-half cups is about the right amount of chopped fruit for an average sized adult to consume in one day.

Kiwi fruit have an added advantage for the eyes. As well as being high in vitamin C, they are also high in lutein and zeaxanthin.[46, 47, 55]

Lutein

Lutein is a powerful antioxidant for eye health, able to fight free radicals and protect cells from oxidative damage. *Lutein is found in green leafy vegetables* like kale and silver beet (sometimes called spinach).

Figure 8: Lutein and Zeaxanthin in Foods

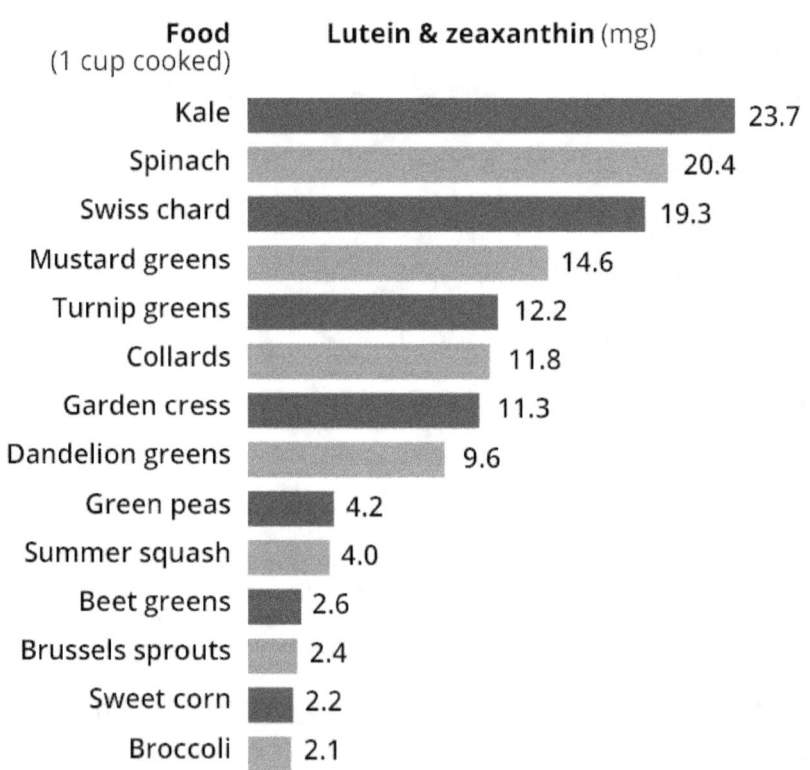

Food (1 cup cooked)	Lutein & zeaxanthin (mg)
Kale	23.7
Spinach	20.4
Swiss chard	19.3
Mustard greens	14.6
Turnip greens	12.2
Collards	11.8
Garden cress	11.3
Dandelion greens	9.6
Green peas	4.2
Summer squash	4.0
Beet greens	2.6
Brussels sprouts	2.4
Sweet corn	2.2
Broccoli	2.1

Source: USDA National Nutrient database for standard reference, 22 (2009).

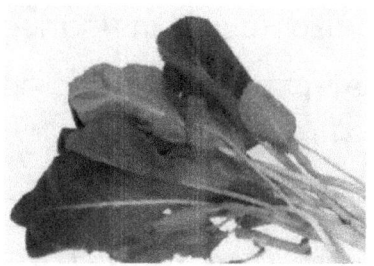

Collards are from the brassica family of plants. They are related to cabbage and are probably Chinese broccoli.

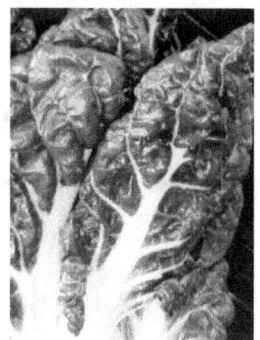

Swiss chard is what Australasians call silver beet or spinach.

Lutein is also in sweet potato, carrots, pumpkin, and other *orange and yellow fruits and vegetables* and orange coloured flowers like marigolds, calendula and nasturtiums – including leaves. These flowers and their leaves are edible and can be used in salads. These all contain excellent antioxidants, which may help protect your eyesight.[54.]

Zeaxanthin

This is one of the most potent antioxidants that we know of to assist our eyes. Like lutein, zeaxanthin is also found in marigolds and kiwi fruit. The by-product, meso-zeaxanthin is normally formed inside our bodies.[48.]

"Lutein and zeaxanthin also work to protect your eyes from free radical damage," says O'Brien.[55.] (My emphasis.)

The table below is another way of looking at the data from the graph on p. 66. Only the vegetables with the highest content are included.

Figure 8: Lutein Content of Green Vegetables

Kale (raw)	26.5
Kale (cooked)	23.4
Spinach (cooked)	20.48
Collards (cooked)	14.6
Turnip greens (cooked)	12.2
Green peas (cooked)	4.1
Spinach (raw)	3.7

"**Mesozeaxanthin** is made by your body from lutein. It can be found in some fish skins, and in supplements containing marigold extract."

Dr. Mosley points out this ingredient may not be listed on some supplement labels.[48.]

Astaxanthins

This group of antioxidants are in the carotenoid group. They are found in orange and red coloured foods, in particular in Pacific salmon and pink seafood (prawns and krill) and the microalgae, *H. pluvialis.* Astaxanthins are unstable and need to be consumed fresh or kept in premium storage conditions.[59] They are the only known antioxidant to cross both the blood brain and blood retinal barriers, reaching tissues important for eye health.[60]

Anthocyanins

Anthocyans are flavonoids - nutrients that are highly valuable for eye health. They are found in the red/purple/blue pigment found in many fruits and vegetables such as:

red cabbage
purple and black carrots
purple cauliflower
red capsicum
blackberries,
blackcurrants
blueberries
mulberries
acai berries
Red and black grapes
Black rice

As well as acting as antioxidants and fighting free radicals, anthocyanins are also believed to be anti-inflammatory, anti-viral, and have anti-cancer benefits.[48, 54, 58, 62]

Blueberries are a very popular fruit and these berries are rich in anthocyanins. The anthocyanins in blueberry may be useful against several chronic diseases including cardiovascular disorders, neurodegenerative diseases, diabetes, cancer and eye diseases.

Whether frozen or fresh, blueberries have one of the highest antioxidant levels among all fruits and may boost memory, the cardiovascular system, and eyesight.

Acai berries are also extremely high in anthocyanins. They grow on acai palm trees in the Amazon rainforest and are processed into a pulp before eating. These are not readily available fresh in Australasia.

More available than acai berries are **black currants**, which are also extremely high in antioxidants including vitamin C. They are a cool climate fruit and most readily available from supermarkets as a dried fruit ingredient used in rich fruit cakes. Beware of brands with added sugar.

Recent and current research from the University of Sydney is emphasising the role of antioxidants from vegetables and fruits in helping prevent eye disorders.[54, 55]

Cathaxanthin

Canthaxanthin belongs to a group of food chemicals called terpenoids. The subgroup is keto-carotenoids; they are found in a kind of wild mushroom. (It is not advisable to experiment with wild mushrooms. Many are toxic.) Many top antioxidants are also found in marine microalgae that fish eat. Hence the importance of farmed fish diets.

Canthaxanthin is created synthetically and added to food products fed to domestically raised chickens, fish and crustaceans, increasing the intensity of yellow in egg yolks and the pink in aquaculture salmon, trout and crustaceans like prawns, crabs, lobster and krill. It is also, in some countries, legal to create tanning products using canthaxanthin.

It is possible that an excess of this synthetic substance will congregate in the retina, producing inflammation in the eye.[32, 59]

Research conducted by Alagawany shows that natural antioxidants, including canthaxanthin, have anti-cancer properties when added to the diet of chickens.[38]

Given that free-range chickens feeding on grasses and grains already have yellow egg yolks, and wild caught Atlantic salmon have pink tones, it is obvious that chickens do consume carotenoids and likewise fish eat algae and krill to give these natural colourings. (Barn raised chickens have carotenoids added to their food.)

Resveratrol

The skins of dark-coloured grapes contain resveratrol. This is part of a group of compounds called polyphenols that act like antioxidants. They protect the body against damage that can put you at higher risk for things like cancer and heart disease, as well as eye disease. [59, 61]

Studies have shown resveratrol in red and black grapes not only penetrates the blood-

brain barrier, but actually helps maintain its integrity.

Resveratrol has been suggested previously as a promoter of health in dry eye, glaucoma, cataracts, age-related macular degeneration (AMD), and diabetic retinopathy.[59, 60]

"...red grapes and concord grapes are higher than sultana grapes in flavonoids and phytonutrients, including resveratrol." (Rumsey reported in Coulston and Bouchey). [34]

Although all types of grapes are healthy in moderation, they are very high in fructose, also known as fruit sugar. Whilst whole fruit is very good for us, too much contains too much sugar, especially when juiced.

Flavonoids

Flavonoids are antioxidants that also contain other nutrients. Foods high in flavonoids are possibly beneficial and protective against AMD and other eye conditions.

Researcher Associate Professor Gopinath, of Sydney University, focused on the relationship between flavonoids and macular degeneration.[58, 59]

She says, "Flavonoids are powerful antioxidants found in almost all fruits and vegetables, and they have important anti-inflammatory benefits for the immune system. We examined common foods that contain flavonoids such as tea, apples, red wine and oranges.

"Significantly, the data did not show a relationship between other food sources protecting the eyes against disease," she said.[58.]

In this chapter, I have drawn on information in Dunn, a text that lists the basic nutrients of most ingredients used in western European diets. [64.]

*

The information and research in this chapter is general in nature. For the most up to date research results about your eye condition, you need to consult your eye practitioner.

Seven

Foods that Help our Eyes

Human beings have developed as omnivorous creatures. A wide range of fresh foods is good for our total body health. Vegetables of as many varieties and as many different colours as possible should be a major part of our diet. Colourful fruits and vegetables contain antioxidants. These are excellent for our general health as well as particularly good for our eyes and brains.

To these, we can add small amounts of fruit (approximately one and a half cupsful per day), raw nuts and seeds. As well, full fat, unflavoured fermented milk products (yoghurt, buttermilk and kefir), butter, cheese, eggs, fish and grass-fed meats also contribute to a healthy diet.

A good diet and plenty of exercise out of doors are ways to ward off all health problems and these include eye problems and the maintenance of good eyesight.[45, 46, 50, 51.]

Best Foods to Help Maintain Healthy Eyes:

These are reputed to be the best foods for your eyes. They are listed in order of potency:

Kiwi, (vitamin C and lutein)

Kale, (lutein, zeaxanthin)

Silver beet (AKA chard) (lutein, zeaxanthin)

Chinese broccoli (AKA collards) (lutein, zeaxanthin)

Blueberries (anthocyanin)

Red cabbage (anthocyanin)

Spinach (lutein, zeaxanthin)

Black currants (anthocyanin)

Oily fish like wild salmon, herring, mackerel, sardines, krill (omega 3 & astaxanthin)

Red and black grapes (resveratrol)

Orange & purple sweet potato (lutein, astaxanthin)

Butternut pumpkin (lutein)

Red capsicum (lutein)

Black rice (anthocyanin)

Grass fed lamb (iron and Essential Fatty Acids including omega 3)

Flowers of nasturtiums, calendula and marigolds (lutein)

Oranges and mandarins (Vitamin C, lutein & other flavonoids)

Oysters (zinc)

Eggs (carotenoids, lecithin, choline)

Wheat germ (vitamin E)

Turkey (vitamin B3, i.e. niacin or nicotinamide)

Unless your food is grown in well-composted soils with a wide range of nutrients from animal and plant sources, without pesticides or concentrated phosphates and nitrates, it will not have as complete a source of nutrients as healthy bodies require.[12, 19, 20, 21 32, 33, 35.]

Moreover, as we age, our bodies require even more nutrients to maintain healthy regeneration of cells. Yet, at the same time, we tend to be cutting back on heavy manual or brainwork and so require less food. How do we gain enough nutrients to maintain our cells?

Most eye doctors tell their patients to eat kale, silver beet and spinach. These will not give up their antioxidants readily. The leaves contain **oxalic acid**, a naturally occurring chemical that prevents the absorption of nutrients.

To get rid of oxalic acid, heat the leaves in water for one minute and then drain. Rinse in fresh water and steam or stir-fry for a few minutes until the leaves soften. This helps break down the cell walls, allowing humans to digest the leaves more easily and make the nutrients more bioavailable.

Supplements

Unless we are growing all our own vegetables in rich soil and without pesticides and weed killers, the only way to maintain our health in retirement and aging is to take high quality supplements.

Pharmaceutical companies like to push the notion that supplements just make expensive urine. And that is true if you take cheap, synthetic vitamins and minerals from the wrong source or in the wrong balance.

There are two ways to approach supplements:

> Do a huge amount of research, study bio-chemistry and learn to read and assess the quality of medical research yourself.

> Or consult a person who has already done this and is a qualified nutritional consultant. Many high quality supplements are available only to practitioners.

Once you know what to look for, it is possible to by-pass the half-knowledge of staff in many health food shops or discount chemists selling a large range of products. Some health food shops employ a fully trained naturopath once or twice a month. It is worthwhile consulting one of these professionals.

Hints

Here are some hints about finding the right supplements that will actually be absorbed by your body and help your eyes.

Vitamins and minerals need to be in the correct dosage and balance to be useful. Too much and too little are both dangerous.

If you are taking pharmaceutical medications, check with the prescribing doctor or your pharmacist whether any particular supplements are contra-indicated.

Vitamins

True vitamins are water-soluble and require only small amounts for normal use. Those who suffer from poor digestion or other gut issues will need to take more.

A. Oil-based vitamin A is good for your skin and beta-carotene for your eyes. The ARED study showed that supplementary beta-carotene was contra-indicated for smokers (and, presumably, for those who had recently stopped smoking). Vitamin A is the preferred supplement for eyes. Your body will convert what it needs to beta-carotene.[63]

B. B vitamins need to be in the correct balance *to be effective. In most instances, it is no use to* take just one B vitamin and ignore the rest. A general multi-vitamin should contain somewhere between 10 and 25 mg of each B1, B2, B3, B6. Take higher levels only if you are extremely stressed. Vitamin B9 is folate, which we find in green leafy vegetables. Supplement with B9 if you have trouble absorbing foods or if you are pregnant. B 12 is found only in eggs and red meats like beef, lamb, goat and kangaroo. Many vegetarians and vegans need to have B12 by injection.

C. A fit person with normal digestion should be able to get sufficient vitamin C from eating freshly picked raw vegetables and fruit. If not, up to 100mg-500mg per day is recommended. For those who are have Irritable Bowel Syndrome, are sick, stressed or anxious, 1-2 grams per day is good unless it provokes diarrhoea. Then you should take less.

D. Vitamin D is an oil-based hormone normally produced by our skin in sunlight. We know it as 'the sunshine vitamin'. As one ages, the skin does not absorb vitamin D so well. A supplement of two oil-based capsules each morning is helpful (2000 International Units) and three capsules in winter. Vitamin D assists with the absorption of minerals (especially calcium and magnesium) into our bones. It also helps retain good mood and a healthy nervous system. (Eight capsules or 16,000 IU is the absolute maximum that one should take without medical supervision.)

E   Vitamin E is not a vitamin either, but an antioxidant which, like vitamins A & D, needs oil or fat to be absorbed. Wheat germ is an important source and you can sprinkle it over cold cereal. Vitamin E is readily destroyed by heat and light. In capsules, it is available in 500 and 1000 IU of d alpha tocopherol. For most of us, 250 IU or less is a sufficient daily dose[46, 47]. The 250 IU product was withdrawn in October 2020 and is no longer sold in Australia.

Too much vitamin E could be detrimental, especially if it is synthetic. Dr M. Lelah says, "Synthetic alpha-tocopherol is only half as active in the body as the natural form. In a review of comparison studies between natural Vitamin E and synthetic Vitamin E in animals and in humans, **natural sourced Vitamin E is at least twice as effective as synthetic** Vitamin E based on physiological and pharmacological markers. There are no good studies comparing the effects of natural Vitamin E vs. synthetic Vitamin E on human diseases.

"In addition, other work presented at this conference indicates that many of the components of natural Vitamin E, gamma-tocotrienol, for example, have their own specific physiological benefits." [51]

K. Vitamin K2 is necessary to assist with the absorption of bone minerals, especially calcium. [65]

Co Q10 This is also known as Vitamin Q, co-enzyme Q10 or ubiquinone. It is an organic molecule similar in structure to vitamin K and vitamin E. Like those, it is also fat-soluble. Co Q10 helps modulate energy production.

Minerals

Minerals work as co-enzymes and catalysts for all sorts of processes in the human body.

The danger with mineral supplements is that they are often contaminated with dangerous heavy metals like mercury, lead and cadmium. This is more likely in cheap supplements derived from low quality sources. Note that too much and too little are dangerous.

The best absorbed minerals come from plant or animal sources, not out of the ground.

The most important minerals to supplement are these:

Calcium and K2 are very important for our bones and nervous system. Calcium also acts as a co-enzyme to activate muscles.[64]

If calcium is not balanced with magnesium and several other bone minerals, it will deposit as spurs on heels and shoulders, and calcifications in joints rather than building bones.

Magnesium Magnesium is a hugely important mineral involved in over 500 hundred bodily processes. Almonds, Brazil nuts and cashews have particularly good levels of magnesium.[59] Most modern humans in western society have a deficiency.

Magnesium (chelate, glycinate or citrate) needs to be balanced with calcium and potassium intake for bone, muscle and cardiovascular health.

Magnesium is a co-enzyme for relaxing our muscles and helps with muscle twitches, restless legs, insomnia and other nervous system ailments. It helps you sleep if you take it at night before bed.

Potassium This mineral is essential for the removal of waste from our cells. It is found in all vegetables, bananas and also tea. We need large amounts. It is poured down the drain if vegetables are boiled and strained. Make a gravy or just drink the cooking water. Potassium needs to be balanced with sodium chloride (common salt) in a ratio of one potassium chloride to two sodium chloride. Potassium takes fluids along with waste products out of our cells into our blood for elimination. It is a natural diuretic.

It is no longer possible to buy the supplement *Slow K* (potassium in a slow release tablet) over the pharmacy counter because it interferes with prescribed diuretics and too much is dangerous. However, there is a supermarket product called Lite Salt, which is half sodium chloride and half potassium chloride. Unfortunately, Lite Salt also contains a large amount of aluminium silicate that is a 'free flow' ingredient. This additive is not good for us.

If you have health issues, it is important to talk to your doctor before using this product.

Sodium Chloride (common salt.) Salt is a necessary mineral that takes nutrient laden fluids into our cells. It is important to have one and a half to two full teaspoons of salt a day. If you cook your own food, you can see how much added salt there is. Processed foods, particularly corned beef, cheese, salted nuts and snacks, often contain too much salt and it is very difficult to estimate how much you are consuming. Always buy iodised salt unless you particularly require non-iodised salt, e.g for the preservation of foods. Only a small percentage of people need to have a restricted intake of sodium salt. Your risk of heart disease is higher if you have more or less than approximately 1.5 – 2.0g of sodium per day.[67] Remember is must be balance with potassium in vegetables.

Iodine This is a very important mineral for your thyroid function. Too little iodine leads to goitre, a swelling on the thyroid and an upset metabolism.

Hence we have *iodised salt*. Industrial food processers tend to use non-iodised salt.

Silica Silica is important for the regeneration of keratin, the protein in hair, skin and fingernails. Insufficient silica leads to brittle nails and hair, and dry flaking skin.

Boron Boron is required in very small amounts. It is found in green leafy vegetables, non-citrus fruits and tree nuts. It is used for building strong bones, treating osteoarthritis, as an aid for building muscles and increasing testosterone levels. It also improves thinking skills and muscle co-ordination.

Chromium This is an important mineral along with vitamin B6. These two nutrients are used in the process of taking carbohydrates (sugars and starches) into our cells. A lack of these nutrients can lead to diabetes. Processing strips these nutrients out of sugars and grains.

Copper was adequately supplied when our water flowed through copper pipes. Copper deficiency is associated with osteoarthritis. Copper must be balanced with zinc and taken separately because they use the same uptake pathway.

Iron provides the red in our red blood cells. It carries the oxygen we need. One or two meals of red meat or eggs in a week provide plenty of iron.

Manganese is another contributor to bone health. Like boron, only small quantities are required.

Sulphur This is found in cruciferous vegetables: cabbage, broccoli, Brussel's sprouts etc., and also in the onion family. It is not usual to supplement with sulphur.

Selenium is widely known to be deficient in Australasian soils and requires supplementation. It is found in imported Brazil nuts. In New Zealand, the health department recommends every person take a supplement of selenium.

Zinc needs to be supplemented before bed, where it can sit in the bowel overnight for optimum absorption.

It is involved in the function of hundreds of enzymes, as well as in cell growth and cell death. Zinc rids the body of dead and unnecessary cells. It assists in detoxification and rids the body of oxidative free radicals and trans-fatty acids.

Zinc also helps our senses of taste and smell. It is very important to consume enough as we age.

Zinc is found naturally in oysters, but there is widespread contamination of these shellfish with heavy metals. Too much zinc is toxic.

These are the major vitamins and minerals required for healthy living. Essential Fatty Acids are the other essential nutrient.

Fish oil Supplements

Omega 3 essential fatty acids contain two important ingredients – EPA (eicosapentaenoic acid) and DHA (docosahexaenoic acid). Their ratio is particularly important when you are choosing a supplement. The normal capsule contains 270:180mg or approximately 5:3 of these two acids.

I am excited to learn from research for this book, that grass fed lamb also contains sufficient omega 3 to be a worthwhile source. We need more research to know about the EPA and DHA levels in lamb. Fresh lamb is a non-inflammatory red meat.

Remember, the body cannot make these nutrients; only fish can by eating algae. That's why they are labelled 'essential'. Only a few people can absorb any from plant sources.[39]

Eight
Blood Supply to your Eyes

The best diet in the world and the best nutrient supplements will not help your eyes if your blood cannot bring those nutrients to your eyes.

Ways to keep your blood moving:

1. **Exercise** such as walking, jogging, cycling, and swimming is the very best way to keep your blood moving so that it brings nutrients to your eyes. Aqua aerobics is good too.

NB: If you suffer from high-pressure glaucoma, keep your head higher than your heart when you exercise.

2. **Acupuncture** can also help blood circulation when the acupuncturist targets the appropriate meridian.

3. **Vibration**: There are platforms that vibrate the entire body from a standing position or by moving your feet while lying down. There are vibrating chairs and vibrating mats which can be laid on a mattress. The latter usually include heating. When your body vibrates, the blood will

move and you will eventually feel your skin itching from the increased circulation. If you cannot walk, cycle or swim, you need to vibrate your body every day so that your circulation takes good nutrients to every part of your body, especially your brain and eyes. Your circulation also removes waste from the body.

4. **Move your eye focus:** make a habit of changing your focus from near to medium distance and to far distance and back again when you are outdoors. Keep the muscles of your eyes active, too.

Nine

In Summary - How to proceed

This chapter gives you a summary of the ways **food and exercise** may help to save your eyesight.

A fit and healthy body is more likely to have healthy eyes. The suggestions made in this book mainly apply to those who are mostly in good health but concerned about preserving their eyesight.

Remember that if you take prescribed medications for serious ailments, it is important to check with your doctor before making major changes to your exercise, diet and taking supplements.

Foods to Eat

Fruit is best for you eaten whole or peeled, but not juiced. Juice releases too many sugars too quickly. A total of approximately one and a half cups of fruit is adequate over one day: Do not cut the fruit up to measure the quantity unless you intend to eat it all in one sitting. Cut fruit will quickly lose its vitamin C and other antioxidant qualities.

Choose from:

Fruits

Berries like blueberries, black berries, mulberries, elderberries (in UK and not readily available in Australasia) and black currants (Tasmania, New Zealand), acai berries (South America) and black, blue or purple grapes.

Kiwi fruit, Papaya, strawberries.

Stone fruit, like black plums, apricots.

Vegetables

Eat at least five servings per day of colourful vegetables. A serving should be half a cup of steamed/cooked vegetables or a cup of raw salad.

Orange and yellow coloured vegetables and plants:

pumpkin

sweet potato (orange/gold or with purple flesh)

carrots

nasturtium, marigold and calendula flowers and leaves

yellow capsicum

corn on the cob

Red/purple/black vegetables

red cabbage

red capsicum

tomatoes

purple sweet potato

purple cauliflower

purple carrots

black (wild) rice

Green Vegetables

kale

broccoli

silver beet

spinach

Chinese greens, especially Chinese broccoli

Brussel's sprouts

green cabbage

green beans

asparagus

avocado

Meats

Lamb preferably grass fed.

Chicken preferably free range on pasture

Turkey preferably free range on pasture.

Fish – especially wild caught, deep-sea fish (salmon, herring, mackerel and sardines (fresh, frozen or canned).

We need proteins from meats, fowl and fish. Keep beef eating as a special treat. It is usually grain fattened with grains from plants that have been drenched in glyphosate weed killers.

Do not rely on tuna for your omega 3 fatty acids. It contains only far less than salmon or even lamb.

Leave the fat on unless it is really excessive. Cooking meat with the fat on increases the flavour.

Remember, research has supported the eating of animal fats for over thirty years. There was no contention about animal foods for thousands of years until processed foods emerged aggressively onto the market and manufacturers saw animal foods as competition.

It is sugars, grains and polyunsaturated seed oils that endanger our health.

Eggs

Free-range eggs are excellent for you. By 'free-range', I mean eggs from those birds allowed to roam on clean pasture, not those that are de-beaked and confined to the floor of a barn. Free-range birds will naturally eat caterpillars, slugs, snails, worms and beetles as well as greens like grass and edible weeds. Poultry should also be fed organically grown, mixed grains. Birds are natural eaters of grains and seeds. Beef cattle and sheep are naturally grass eaters.

For most people, two or three eggs per day are a healthy addition to your diet. The idea that eggs contain cholesterol that will raise the level of your blood cholesterol was scotched by nutritional researchers decades ago. This is yet another piece of misinformation perpetuated via the drug companies and the medical fraternity. If you do not eat enough cholesterol, your body will produce it for you.

Warning for those with Autoimmune Disorders

Some plant foods contain natural chemicals designed to deter critters, including humans, from eating them. These natural chemicals are salicylic acids, commonly referred to as salicylates (eg asprin); some also contain amines (free amino acids) and glutamates (often in Chinese food), and some, like tomatoes, contain all three.

Many people with autoimmune disorders are sensitive to these naturally occurring chemicals as well as to other laboratory-manufactured chemicals that are added to food. Symptoms can include fatigue, hyperactivity, inability to concentrate, muscle aches and pains, nerve and gut irritability. (See The Royal Prince Alfred Guide to low chemical foods.[68.])

It *is* possible to find enough fresh fruits and vegetables with high levels of antioxidants to protect your eyes even if you have to avoid some other varieties. I know from personal experience.

Cooking

The safest ways to cook your foods and avoid potential disease is to steam, poach or simmer on the stovetop. Remember to get rid of the oxalic acid from your leafy greens by bringing them to the boil, rinsing and re-steaming them.

You can cook vegetables in the microwave, but do not cook meats, fish or eggs that way. Microwaves do not heat the food evenly and can heat small areas of food to a very high temperature, destroying the structure of the natural fatty acids and turning them into carcinogenic trans-fatty acids. You can thaw frozen food in your microwave; just make sure the settings are low so the food cannot over-heat. Barbecuing food raises the risk of burning fats. Try to find ways to use your barbecue that do not char your food.

Avoid over-heating oils and fats. Add water before heating. Discard oil that has smoked and burnt. Trim off burnt fat from barbequed and char-grilled meats. Make a barbeque a treat.

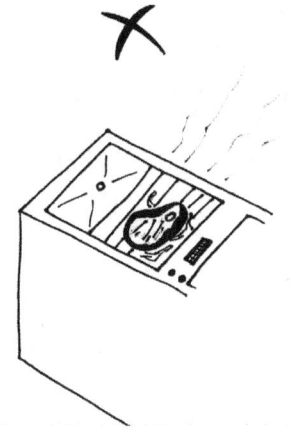

Avoid char-grilled meat and burnt fat

Supplements Recommended for Eye Health

The most necessary supplements for your eyes are antioxidants. Oxidative stress is involved in many eye diseases, but especially macular degeneration. The AREDs (Age Related Eye Diseases Study) started collecting data in 1998. It was originally planned to collect data about AMD and cataract development.[63.]

In 2013, a second study was undertaken because the nutrients recommended on the basis of the first study were inadequate for many people. Smokers were found to be at higher risk of lung cancer when they took 15 mg beta carotene per day. AREDS recommend vitamin A instead.

The AREDS2 study came up with the following recommendation for daily dietary supplementation:[57.]

Zinc (oxide)	80 mg
Vitamin C	500 mg
Vitamin E	400 IU
Copper (Cupric Oxide)	2 mg
Lutein	10 mg
Zeaxanthin	2 mg

Note that the Macular Disease Foundation makes no recommendation for the kind of tocopherol used in the vitamin E supplement.

I highly recommend **d alpha tocopherol** and gamma tocopherol. Synthetic (dl) vitamin E might be harmful. I also recommend a lower dose of zinc.

"...d-alpha tocopherol is only one of the eight naturally occurring plant constituents. Vitamin E also contains three other tocopherol isomers – beta, delta, and gamma. There are also four active tocotrienols, which have powerful antioxidant capabilities. The majority of nutritional supplements are stripped not only of the other three active tocopherols but also the tocotrienols. Additionally, gamma tocopherol is the superior tocopherol of the four," says Dr. Stephen Gangemi, of North Carolina.[51.]

For those who have one or more degenerative eye diseases, I suggest the following daily supplements:

Antioxidants:
- A (1000 IU) or equivalent in beta carotene for non-smokers
- C (500mg +)
- D 2000 – 5000 IU
- E (d alpha tocopherol) 250 IU (or 500 IU every second day)

> Zinc (25-30mg)
>
> Lutein (2mg)
>
> Zeanthaxin (10mg)
>
> Astaxanthin (4 - 12 mg)

A good mineral supplement, well-balanced with calcium (citrate or hydroxyapatite), magnesium (chelate, citrate or glycinate), potassium (chloride) and sodium (chloride) will assist with blood pressure, glaucoma and cataracts. A soup base made from boiled lamb shank or chicken bones (free range) contains good minerals too. Remove the bones when the water has cooled.

B vitamins: 10mg of each B vitamin is normally sufficient unless you are working in a highly stressful situation when 25mg or even 50mg might be needed. B vitamins must be in the correct ratio.

Cautionary Note: Slow release supplements might not dissolve in the gut of an older person. These are best avoided if you have any digestive issues or if you are over 65.

B vitamins are usually synthetic. I have just heard before going to press about natural B vitamins now being made in Germany from sprouted quinoa seeds. Keep a look out for these products reaching our shores.

Exercise gets the nutrients from these important foods and supplements into your arteries, heart, brain, and eyes.

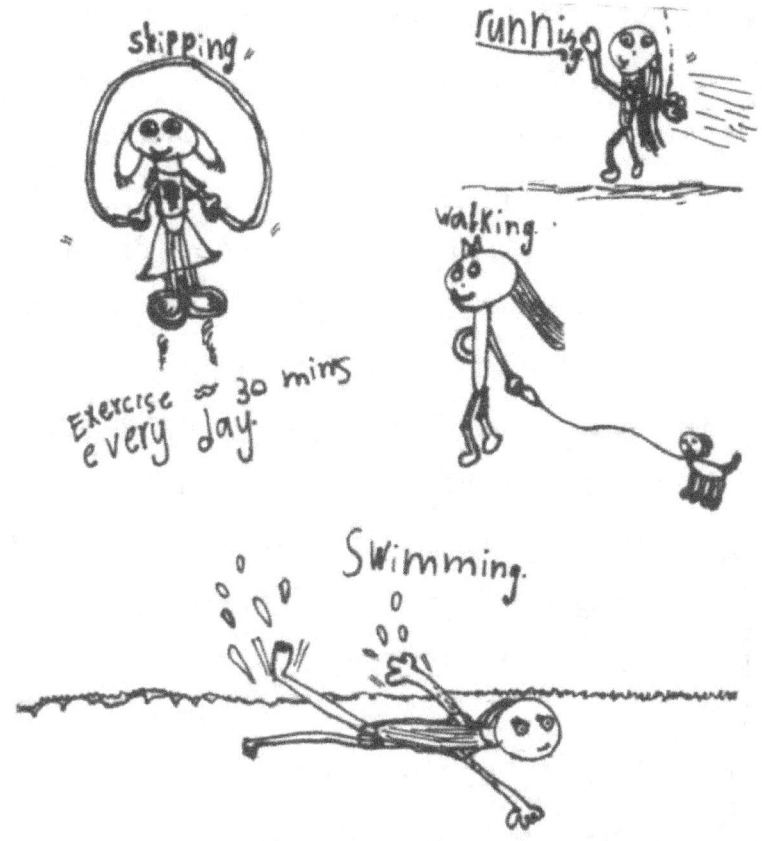

Skipping, running, walking and swimming are all excellent ways to exercise and move your blood and nutrients

Gardening is excellent exercise for those who are able. Bending to weed and plant, and lawn mowing are good for those who are more fit. Minimum exercise is to walk for half an hour every day. Housework also helps us keep fit, especially sweeping, using a vacuum cleaner and hanging out washing. Having a dog is a great incentive to walk. Alternatively, cycle or swim for half an hour. A stationary bicycle is excellent for older people who are prone to falling off. If you are unable to walk but have reasonable balance, use a vibration platform for ten minutes twice a day, or one that moves your legs while you are lying on the floor or on a bed. Otherwise, use a machine that enables you to sit and move your legs in a cycling motion or even a foot vibrator. Full body massage also gets the blood moving. Discuss your proposed exercise regime with your general practitioner before you start anything vigorous.

~

I realise that what I am suggesting might entail considerable adaptation to your normal daily routines regarding foods and exercise. It depends what you want to achieve as to how motivated you will be.

Even small changes in the right direction will be beneficial.

For some, it will be better to change everything all at once. For others, small changes over a period of time will work better. It is your health and for you to decide what works best for you.

For some of you, it might involve learning to cook! This will be easier to do if you are retired or work part-time. Treat it as a fun exercise and see how much better the food will taste. It will work out cheaper too, yet better quality. Full-time workers could cook at the weekend and freeze foods for nights when you will be too tired to cook.

If there is no stove or cooker where you live, you can buy a cheap plug-in hot plate at a hardware store. Thaw your cooked and frozen food on a plate over a saucepan of boiling water.

See your Dentist

Oral health care is vital. The most recent research on micro-organisms in our mouths shows a link between gum disease like gingivitis, periodontal disease and root canals to many inflammatory and degenerative disorders, including heart disease and macular degeneration.[27.]

*

If you follow my recommendations, you may well be able to slow down or prevent eye disease as I have and, I hope, maintain your eyesight for many years to come.

Acknowledgements

I want to acknowledge ophthalmologist, Dr. Peter Davies of the Newcastle Eye Hospital, for suggesting that I write this book. It has taken me several years to act on his suggestion.

Credit goes to my very good friend, Dr. Judith Handlinger (retired veterinary pathologist), for pointing out that my first draft was very far from what was needed. She has carefully edited the my referencing method, especially of on-line journal articles. Judy remained an academic while I became a round the world sailor, teacher, natural therapist and now, author.

My grandchildren, Tane and Kira Mitchell put their hearts into drawing the illustrations Nana asked for. They are delightful and were only finished because of the persistence of their mother, Lisa Herring.

Nick Handlinger made the cover and its illustrations. Thank you Nick. We struggled but, in the end, we achieved a beautiful cover.

The Lake Macquarie branch of the Fellowship of Australian Writers provides huge support and friendship. I also acknowledge Katharina Prior, a member of my writing support group, who suffered from severe vison problems prior to a cataract operation. She is the sort of person I have written this book for and she has given very positive feedback on my choice of script, size of font and the readability of the text.

As always, my husband and sons and their partners are supportive of my writing and publishing. Thank you all.

References

1. Lenscrafters website. "Parts of the eye," https://www.lenscrafters.ca/lc-ca/vision-guide/parts-of-the-eye

2. Harvard Health Newsletter. (2010). "Warning signs of serious eye disease," https://www.health.harvard.edu/diseases-and-conditions/warning-signs-of-a-serious-eye-problem 2010

3. *Fine, Laura. (2018)* "Considering cataract surgery? What you should know." Harvard Women's Health Watch, September, 2016. Updated July 12, 2018

4. Robb-Nicholson, Celeste MD. (2018) "By the way, Doctor, What can I do to prevent cataracts?" Harvard Health Newsletter, July, 2018 https://www.health.harvard.edu/newsletter_article/what-can-i-do-to-prevent-cataracts

5. Mayo Clinic. "Type 2 Diabetes: Symptoms and causes." https://www.mayoclinic.org/diseases-conditions/type-2-diabetes/symptoms-causes/syc-20351193

6. Wachler, Brian MD. reviewer for webmd, (2019) "Dry eyes: home remedies," https://www.webmd.com/eye-health/dry-eyes-home-remedies#1

7. Vision Australia. (2020) "Eye conditions: glaucoma," https://www.visionaustralia.org/

information/eye-conditions/glaucoma

8. Bright Focus website. "Blood pressure and glaucoma," https://www.brightfocus.org/glaucoma/article/blood-pressure-and-glaucoma

9. Seltman, Whitney, reviewer for WebMD. (2019) "Eye Stroke: Causes, Symptoms, and Treatment," September 06, 2019. https://www.webmd.com/eye-health/occular-hypertension#1

10. Mayo Clinic. "Dry macular: symptoms and causes," https://www.mayoclinic.org/diseases-conditions/dry-macular-degeneration/symptoms-causes/syc-20350375

11. Dunaief, Joseph. (2019) "What is Geographic Atrophy?" https://www.brightfocus.org/macular/article/what-geographic-atrophy updated 2019

12. Francis, Raymond and King, Michelle. (2007) "Never Be Fat Again," Health Communications Inc, Florida."

13. Chao-Wen Lin, et al. (2019) "The effects of reflected glare and visual field lighting on computer vision syndrome," Clin Exp Optom., Sep;102(5):513-520. https://pubmed.ncbi.nlm.nih.gov/30805993

14. Aurora Healthcare website. (2018) "Why Sunshine is Good for Your Vision," https://www.aurorahealthcare.org/services/eye-care

15. Golan, D. et. al. (2013) "The influence of vitamin D supplementation on melatonin status in patients with multiple sclerosis", Brain, Behavior, and Immunity. Golan-Staun-ram/e844c00e875bc24bb2cd184f460c7807d23382a7

16. Rose , Kathryn A. et al. (2008) "Myopia, Lifestyle, and Schooling in Students of Chinese Ethnicity in Singapore and Sydney." Arch Ophthalmol. April 1, 2008;126(4):527-530 (doi:10.1001/archopht.126.4.527).

17. Golan, D. et al. (2013) "Multiple sclerosis (MS) incidence is higher in geographic regions with less sunlight exposure," https://www.sciencedirect.com/science/article/abs/pii/S0889159113001785?dgcid=api_sd_search-api-endpoint

18. Healthline. (2015). Carotid Artery Disease," https://www.healthline.com/health/carotid-artery-disease 2015

19. Erasmus, Udo. (1993). "Fats that Heal and Fats that Kill," 2nd edition, Alive Books 1993, Canada.

20. Bredesen, Dr. Dale. (2017) The end of Alzheimers: "The first program to prevent and reverse cognitive decline," P. 48. Vermillion, London.

21. Health Engine website. "Physical Exercise and eye health," https://healthengine.com.au/info/physical-exercise-and-eye-health

22. Healthline website. "Eye exercises," https://www.healthline.com/health/eye-health/eye-exercises

23. ANZ Food Authority. (2001)."Food derived from glyphosate tolerant cotton line 1445: a safety assessment," Technical report series no. 6 Australia New Zealand Food Authority November 2001.

24. Barber, Laurie in "Systemic Drugs with Ocular Side Effects," Review of Ophthalmology, 4 October 2011.

25. Knobbe, Chris A and Stojanoska, Marija. (2017) "The 'Displacing Foods of Modern Commerce' Are the Primary and Proximate Cause of Age-Related Macular Degeneration: A Unifying Singular Hypothesis," Medical Hypotheses Volume 109, November 2017, Pages 184-198.

26. Aminov, Rustam. (2013), "Archaeal microbiota population in piglet feces shifts in response to weaning," www.ncbi.nlm.nih.gov ›

27. MacKenzie, Debora. (2019) "The Hidden Cause of Disease" New Scientist, 10 August pp42-46.

28. Nischwitz, Dr. Dominic. (2019), "It's All in Your Mouth", translated into English by Holly James, 2020, Chelsea Green Publishing, London.

29. Fowler, Paige. "Could My Medications Affect my Sight?" https://www.webmd.com/eye-health/features/medications-cause-vision-problems#1.

30. Stephenson, Michelle. "Systemic Drugs with Ocular Side Effects" Contributing Editor, Review of Ophthalmology, 4 October 2011.

31. Fraunfelder, F. (2011). "Drug induced ocular side effects" Review of Opthalmology, 4 October 2011. https://doi.org/10.1111/j.1442-9071.1984.tb01186.x

32. Robert A. Beaulieu et al. (2013) "Canthaxanthin Retinopathy with Visual Loss: A Case Report and Review" Case Reports in Ophthalmological Medicine October 2013. DOI: 10.1155/2013/140901 Source: Pub Med.

33. Collman, James P. Professor of Chemistry, Stanford University. (2001) "Naturally Dangerous: Surprising Facts about Food, Health, and the Environment," University Science Books, Stanford.

34. Coulston, Ann M., and Boushey, Carol J. Editors, (2008) "Nutrition in the Prevention and Treatment of Disease" Section II, pp 289 – 300. Elsevier Academic Press, USA.

35. Shephard, G.S. (2018) "Aflatoxins in peanut oil: food safety concerns," https://www.wageningenacademic.com/doi/abs/10.3920/WMJ2017.2279

36. Singh, A. (2018) "Cancer! Roots in our Foods," Gut Gastroenterol 2 Volume 1(1): 2018.

37. Mayne, S.T. and Parker, R.S. (1989) "Antioxidant activity of dietary canthaxanthin," Nutr Cancer;12(3):225-36.

38. Alagawany, Mahmoud et. al. (2019) "Omega-3 and Omega-6 Fatty Acids in Poultry Nutrition: Effect on Production Performance and Health," Animals (Basel) 2019 Aug; 9(8): 573. Published online 2019 Aug 18. doi: 10.3390/ani9080573

39. McNally, Janet. (2015) "Land salmon? Grassfed lamb's omega 3 shine," Graze Magazine, March 2015. No Bull Press. www.grazeonline.com › landsalmon

40. Cougnard-grégoire, A et al. (2016) "Olive Oil Consumption and Age-Related Macular Degeneration: The Alienor Study," PLoS One. 2016; 11(7): e0160240. Published online 2016 Jul 28. doi:10.1371/journal.pone.0160240. PMID: 27467382.

41. Wick, Ashley. Reporter on A current Affair, (2020) "Round Up heading to court over cancer claims."

42. Lane, K. (2014) "Bioavailability and Potential Uses of Vegetarian Sources of Omega-3 Fatty Acids: A Review of the Literature," Food Sci Nutr. 2014; 54(5):572-9. https://www.researchgate.net/publication/258827155

43. Embuscado, Milda E. in "Handbook of Antioxidants for Food Preservation." 2015.

44. Kink, Rachel. (2019) "What is Hydrogenated Vegetable Oil?" Healthline, September 2019.
45. Riaz, Mian N. & Rokey, Galen J. (2012) "Extrusion Problems Solved," 2012 Culinary Nutrition, Science Direct 2013.

46. Adela Mariana, et al. (2014) in "Handbook of Nutrition, Diet and the Eye," (ed. Victor R. Preedy) Kings College, London

47. Macula Disease Foundation of Australia website. "Nutrition." https//:www.mdfoundation.com.au/nutrition

48. Mosely, Dr Michael. "Can eating the right foods improve your eyesight? BBC Medical Journalist Believes Certain Foods May Help Eyesight." https://www.vision-care.co.uk/can-eating-the-right-foods-improve-your-eyesight

49. Everything Zoomer website. (2019). "7 Foods to nourish your eyes," www.everythingzoomer.com <2019/05/21 > foods-boost-eye-health 2019

50. Gangemi, Dr. D. "Vitamin E: What you need to know," https://www.drgangemi.com/health-articles/diet-nutrition/vitamin-e-what-you-need-to-know/

51. Lelah, Dr M. (2008) "Natural versus synthetic vitamin E," National Health Research Institiute, July 2, 2008.

52. Hanssen, Maurice and Marsden, Jill. (1989) "The new Additive Code Breaker," Revised by Betty Norris for Australia, Lothian Publishing, Melbourne.

53. Dengate, Sue. (1998) "Fed Up: Understanding How Food Affects Your Child and What You Can Do About It," Random House, NSW, Australia.

54. Ingkasupart, Pajaree et al. (2020) "Antioxidant activities and lutein content of 11 marigold cultivars

(Tagetes.spp.) grown in Thailand," Food Sci. Technol, Campinas, 35(2): 380-385, Apr-Jun.2020.

55. O'Brien, Sharon. (2018) Lutein and Zeaxanthin: Benefits, Dosage and Food Sources."
https://www.healthline.com/nutrition/lutein-and-zeaxanthin, July 11, 2018.

56. Miller ER, et al (2005) "Meta-analysis: high-dosage vitamin E supplementation may increase all-cause mortality,". Annals of Internal Medicine,
 January 2005142 (1): 37–46. (doi:10.7326/0003-4819-142-1-200501040-00110. PMID 15537682).

57. Gopinath, Bamini. (2013) "Is quality of diet associated with the microvasculature? An analysis of Diet Quality and Retinal Vascular calibre in Older Adults," The British journal of nutrition, 110(4):1-8·March 2013.

58. Gopinath, Bamini et al. (2018) "Dietary flavonoids and the prevalence and 15-y incidence of age-related macular degeneration," The American Journal of Clinical Nutrition, Vol. 108, Issue 2, pp 381–387, August 2018.

59. Palozza, P. and Krinsky. N.I.(1992) "Astaxanthin and Canthaxanthin are potent Antioxidants in a Membrane Model," Arch Biochem Biophys, 1992 Sep; 297 (2) 291 – 5
60. Yamashita, Eiji. (2015). "Let Astaxanthin be they medicine," PharmaNutrition 3 (2015) 115–122, Elsevier.

61. Chu, Will. (2017)."Reservatrol and the human retina." www.nutraingredients.com/Article// Resveratrol2017/03/23

62. Szalay, Jessie. (2016) "Grapes: Health Benefits & Nutrition Facts," Live Science, April 28, 2016.
63. Herndon, Jaime R. (2019). "AREDS and AREDS2 Supplements for Macular Degeneration," MD Foundation editorial Team. Reviewed April 2020.

64. Dunn, Lavon J. (2001) "Nutrition Almanac." fifth edition, 183-196. McGraw Hill, Sydney. Published online 2016 Jul 28. doi:10.1371/journal.pone.0160240 PMCID: PMC4965131

65. Eske, Jamie. (2019) "What to Know about Vitamin K1 and K2," Medical News Today, April 2019.

66. Shruti Dighe, et al. (2019) "Diet patterns and the incidence of age-related macular degeneration in Atherosclerosis risk communities (ARIC) study," British Journal of Ophthalmology, 2019-314813 (DOI: 10.1136/bjophthalmol-2019-314813)

67. Hooper L, et al. 2004) "Advice to reduce dietary salt for prevention of cardiovascular disease," Cochrane Database of Systematic Reviews 2004, Issue 1. Art. No.: CD003656. DOI: 10.1002/14651858.CD003656.pub2

68. Swain, Dr. Anne et al. (2016) "Friendly Food: The essential guide to managing common food allergies and intolerances," Royal Prince Alfred Hospital Allergy Unit, Murdoch Books, Sydney, Revised and reprinted 2004. Reprinted 2016.

Index

Acai   69, 70.

Acupuncture   89.

Additive Code Breaker   57, 110.

Aflatoxins`   33, 108.

Aging   8, 15, 23, 60, 78.

Algae   35, 51, 52, 72.

ALA (alpha linolenic acid) 52.

AMD (Age Related Macular Degeneration) 7. **11-12**, 58, 59, 73, 97, 115.

Amines 88, 95.

Anthocyans .69.

Antioxidants 8, 55, **58-60**, 67, 69ff, 77, 96f, 97, 99, 109, 111.

    Natural 29, 48, **57**ff, 60, 63, 67, 99.

    Synthetic 5, 52, 53, 58, **59**ff, 45.

Archaea 24, 25, 42.

Astaxanthins 69.

Autoimmune disorders 59, 95, 101.

Blood 2, 9, 12, 22, 84, 86, 101.

Blood brain barrier 72.

Blood thinners 26, 28, 65 .

Blood Pressure 11, 23, 26, 35, 99.

Calories (kilojoules)   115.

Cancer .19, 35, 39, 46, 47, 53, 60, 64, 70, 72, 98,108,109.

Cardiovascular disease 21, 46, 62, 72.

Carotenes 57f, 79f.

Cataract **6ff**, 21, 23, 29, 73, 97, 100, **103.**

Canthaxanthin 27, 67, 60, 71ff, 107f,111.

Cornea 2.

Cotton bud 10.

Cottonseed 21, 32, 46.

Deep Relaxation 11.

Diabetes **8ff**, 30, 35, 46, 59, 70, 86, 103

DHA & EPA 36, 52, 88.

Diet 7, 9, 10, 13, 14, 20, 23, 33, **34ff,** 43ff 48, 74, 75, 89, 98, 108f, 110ff.

Drinking alcohol 8.

Drugs (also see medicine) iv, 7, 8, 10, 23, 26f, 28, 106, 116.

Drusen 11, 58.

Dry AMD 11, 12.

Dry eye 10, 25.

Electrons 3, **54f,**

Exercise 5, 15, **21ff**, 75, 89, 90, **91,100ff**, **106**

Eye pressure 8.

Eyesight 6, 9, 15f, 18, 29, 102

Fats 3, **23**ff, 37,

    Animal fats. 12, **32ff**, **37**,

    Hydrogenated fat. **39ff**, 46ff, 48, 50

    Trans Fats **53ff**, 58, 94, 97, 106.

Fatty acids **53**.

    Essential fatty acids. 32, 34, 37, 40, 42, 44, 45, 48, 50, 76, 88.

    Omega 3 & omega 6 21, **32ff,** 42, 45, 48ff, 76, 88, 109.

    Fish 28, 32, 34, **35**, 36, 49f, 68, 71, 72, 88, 93, 94, 96.

    Herring 50, 76, 93.

    Krill 36, 50, 69, 71, 72, 76.

    Mackerel 35, 50, 76, 93.

    Salmon **35ff**, 37, 39, 60, 69, 71, 72, 76, 93.

    Tuna 32, 50, 58, 84, 94.

Fish Oils. 28, 32, 36, **49**.

Flavonoids 69, **73**, 74, 76.

Food - Fresh 10, 60, 65, 69, 70, 75, 92, 93, 96.

Food – Processed 12, 20, 21, 29ff, 33, 45, 49, 55, 57, **59**, 70, 85, 94.

Focus 2, 3, 5, 17, 22, 73, 90, 103.

Free Radicals 55, 66, 87.

Genetics 13, 23, 42, 45, 46.

Geographic atrophy 12.

Glare 5, 6, 13, **19**, 23 .

Glaucoma. **11**, 23, 29, 73, 100, 103.

Glucose syrup 21, 29.

Glyphosate 21, 33, 46, 47.

H. pluvialis 69.

High blood pressure 11, 23, 35.

Hormone therapy 8.

Hunter-gatherers 34, 44.

Hydrogenated fat 39.

Hypertensive retinopathy 11.

Immune system 15, 16, 59, 73, 95.

Inflammation 13, 20, 21, **24,** 27, 30, 31, 33, 35, 71.

Iris 1, 2, 5.

Iron 13, 42, 53, 76, 86.

Kilojoules (calories) 41, 43, 44.

Krill 36, 50, 69, 71, 72.

Lens 1, 2, 3, **6f**f, 17.

Light **2ff** 5, 6, 16, 17, 19, 33, 40, 41, 47, 52, 54, 80, 81. 104, 105.

Lipids (see fats & oils) 47, 52, 54, 55.

Lipid peroxidation 55.

Lutein **8f**, 57, 60, **66ff,** 76, 98, 99.

Macula 1, 3,

Macular degeneration 11, **12,** 13, 15, 21, 25, 29, 40, 46, 58, 59, 73, 97, 98, 102, 104.

Mayonnaise 36.

Marine algae 51, 69, 71

Margarine 36, **52**.

Meat 39, 75, 80, 86, **93f**, 96, 97.
    Beef 37, 38, 80, 94, 95.
    Chicken 37, 93, 100.
    Lamb **37f**, 45, 76, 80, 88, 93, 100.
    Pork 37.

Medicare 24.

Medication (also see drugs)10, 17, **25f**, 79, 91.
    Herbal medications **25ff.**

Melatonin 16, 18.

Mezo-zeaxanthin 59.

Microalgae *H. pluvialis* 69.

Microwave cooking. 52, 53.

Minerals 30, 54, 78, 81, **82ff,** 88.
    Boron 86.
    Calcium **7,** 23, 30, **81ff**, 99.
    Chromium. 30, 86.
    Copper 86, 98.
    Iodine 85.
    Iron 13, 42, **53**, 76, 86.

Magnesium 81, **83**, 99.

Manganese 87.

Potassium **83f**, 99.

Silica 85, 86.

Sodium **84-85**.

Sulphur 25, 87.

Zinc 30f, 45, 57, 60, 76, **86ff**.

Mirror image 27, 57, 61.

Mobile phone screens 19.

Molecules 3, 7, 9, 47, 48, **52ff,** 61.

Mould in bread 60.

Mushrooms, wild 27, 71.

Nutritional supplements 9, 10, 13, 18, 26, 28, 32, 35, 49, 57, 61, 64, 68, **78f,** 83, 88f, 91, 97, 99, 100.

Nuts 34, 41, 64, 7, 60ff 75, 83, 85ff.

Obesity 20, 29, 35, 46.

Oils

Avocado 40, 48, 93.

Canola 21, 36, 46.

Coconut 37, 46, 47.

Cooking 7, 21, 37, 41, 45, 46, 52, 65, 84, 94.

Fish oils 32, 36.

Flaxseed 36.

    Hemp 36, 52.

    Krill 36, 50, 69, 71, 72.

    'Lite' oil 41.

    Olive **40,** 48f.

    Mono-saturated **40,** 41, **48.**

    Saturated 37, **47f.**

    Polyunsaturated 32, 41, **49f,** 94.

    Seed oils 10, 20, 32ff, 36, 45, 46, 49, 50.

    Soy 21, 29, **31-32.**

    Sunflower 21, 32, 36.

    Vegetable 12, 21, 32.

    Walnut 40, 48.

Omega 3 & omega 6 fatty acids 21, **32ff,** 42, 45, 48ff, 76, 88, 109

Ophthalmologist 2, 7.

Optic nerve 3.

Optometrist 5, 46.

Osteoporosis. 7.

Oxalic acid 77, 96.

Oxygen 11, 22, 41, 47ff, 52, 54, 57, 86.

Oxidation 39, 52, 54, **55,** 57, 60.

Oxidative rancidity 54.

Plastics 33, 47.

    Micro-plastics 33.

Phospholipids 55.

Phytochemicals 9.

Polyphenols 72.

Processed Food 12, 20, 21, 29ff, 33, 45, 49, 55, 57, **59**, 70, 85, 9412, 59

Pupil 1, 2, 3.

Rancidity 39, 41, **52,** 54.

Refined flour, sugar etc. 10, 29, 30, 31, 35.

Reservatrol 72, 73.

Retina 1, 2, **3**, 11, 17, 27, 71.

Rods and cones 2,3.

Round-up (Glyphosate) 21, 33 46, 47.

Salmon **35ff**, 37, 39, 60, 69, 71, 72, 76, 93.

Sclera 2.

Screens **19**, 22.

Seed oil industry 12, 32, 45, 52.

Sleep 10, 17, 18, 84.

Serving size 92.

Smoking 8, 13, 15, 79.

Smoke point 37, 68.

Sugar (white) 9, 10, 12, 20, 21, **29-31,** 35, 42, 71, 73, 81, 94.

    Dextrose 29.

    Fructose 29.

    Glucose 9, 21, 29, 31.

Maltose 29.

Sucrose 29, 31.

Sunbathing 17.

Sunglasses 8, 20.

Sunscreen 17.

Sunlight 2, 8, **16ff**.

Supplements 9, 10, 13, 18, 26, 28, 32, 35, 49, 57, 61, 64, 68, **78f,** 83, 88f, 91, 97, 99, 100.

Synthetic antioxidants 29, 53, **57,** 59.

Tocopherols

    d alpha tocopherol 61, 63, 81, 98, 99.

    dl alpha tocopherol 61.

    gamma tocopherol 63ff, 65, 82, 98, 99.

VDTs (Video display terminals) 13.

Vibration 98, 101.

Vitamins 9, 30, 57, 60, 61, 63, 71, 78, **79,** 80, 88, 100.

    A 79, 80.

    Bs. 30, 76, 80.

    C 65, 66, 76, 80, 91, 98.

    D 16, 18, 81.

    E 28, 31, **60-65**, 76, **81**f, 98.

    K2 82, 83.

    Q10. 82.

Wet AMD 12.

WWII 31, 46.

Zeaxanthin 9, 57, 60, 66, **67f,** 76, 98

About the Author

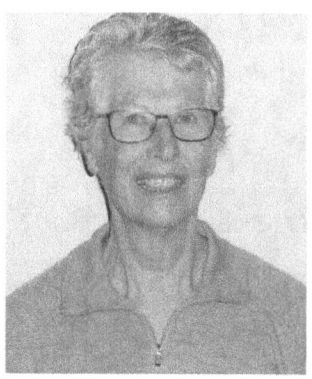

Jan Mitchell grew up in New Zealand and now lives with her husband beside beautiful Lake Macquarie in NSW, Australia.

She has enjoyed writing both creatively and in non-fiction since her early teens. Much of her adult published writing has been in the form of magazine articles for *Cruising Helmsman*, a magazine for cruising yachtsmen and women.

Jan has published four nonfiction books, the first a biography of a friend (**tinker, tailor, soldier, sailor – the life of Colin Kerby OAM**) and then a three-volume memoir of her forty years of ocean cruising. In the latter, she included most of the already published sailing articles she'd written over the years.

She followed that up with a couple of storybooks for her beloved grandchildren.

More lately has been honing her skills in fictional short story writing. She has been commended in two short story writing competitions.

As JB Mitchell, she now also writes about nutrition. **Food for Eyes** is her first book in the *Food for …* series.

***

Notes

978-0-6484976-4-6
Imprint: Lakehouse Publishing